Textbook of

Herbal
Cosmetics

Textbook of
Herbal
Cosmetics

M. Vimaladevi
BSc, MPharm, PhD

Emeritus Professor of Pharmaceutical Technology
Andhra University
Visakhapatnam, AP

Honorary Chairperson
Auro Pharma
Puducherry

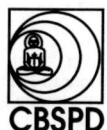

CBSPD

CBS Publishers & Distributors Pvt Ltd

New Delhi • Bengaluru • Chennai • Kochi • Kolkata • Lucknow • Mumbai
Hyderabad • Jharkhand • Nagpur • Patna • Pune • Uttarakhand

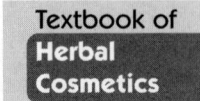

Textbook of
Herbal
Cosmetics

ISBN: 978-81-239-2502-8

First Edition: 2015
Reprint 2017, 2019, 2022

Published by Satish Kumar Jain and produced by Varun Jain for

CBS Publishers & Distributors Pvt Ltd
4819/XI Prahlad Street, 24 Ansari Road, Daryaganj, New Delhi 110 002, India
Ph: 011-23289259, 23266861, 23266867   Website: www.cbspd.com
Fax: 011-23243014   e-mail: delhi@cbspd.com; cbspubs@airtelmail.in
Corporate Office: 204 FIE, Industrial Area, Patparganj, Delhi 110 092
Ph: 011-4934 4934   Fax: 011-4934 4935   e-mail: publishing@cbspd.com; publicity@cbspd.com

Branches

- **Bengaluru:** Seema House 2975, 17th Cross, K.R. Road, Banasankari 2nd Stage, Bengaluru 560 070, Karnataka, India
  Ph: +91-80-26771678/79   Fax: +91-80-26771680   e-mail: bangalore@cbspd.com
- **Chennai:** 7, Subbaraya Street, Shenoy Nagar, Chennai 600 030, Tamil Nadu, India
  Ph: +91-44-26680620, 26681266   Fax: +91-44-42032115   e-mail: chennai@cbspd.com
- **Kochi:** 42/1325, 1326, Power House Road, Opp KSEB, Power House, Ernakulam 682 018, Kerala, India
  Ph: +91-484-4059061-65   Fax: +91-484-4059065   e-mail: kochi@cbspd.com
- **Kolkata:** 147, Hind Ceramics Compound, 1st Floor, Nilgunj Road, Belghoria, Kolkata-700056, West Bengal, India
  Ph: 033-25633055, 033-25633056   e-mail: kolkata@cbspd.com
- **Lucknow:** Basement, Khushnuma Complex, 7-Meerabai Marg (Behind Jawahar Bhawan) Lucknow 226001, India
  Ph: 0522-4000032   e-mail: tiwari.lucknow@cbspd.com
- **Mumbai:** PWD Shed. Gala no. 25/26, Ramchandra Bhatt Marg, Next to JJ Hospital Gate no. 2, Opp. Union Bank of India, Noorbaug Mumbai-400009, Maharashtra, India
  Ph: 022-66661880/89   e-mail: mumbai@cbspd.com

Representatives

- **Hyderabad** 0-9885175004   • **Jharkhand** 0-9811541605   • **Nagpur**   0-9421945513
- **Patna**   0-9334159340   • **Pune**   0-9623451994   • **Uttarakhand** 0-9716462459

Printed at SRK Graphics, Delhi, India

to

*the Mother
and
Sri Aurobindo*

and

Late Prof R.V. Krishna Rao
eminent phytochemist and pharmacognosist

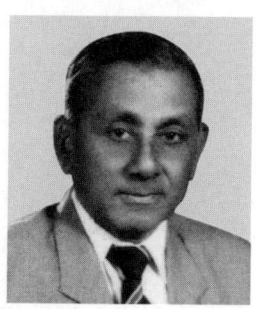

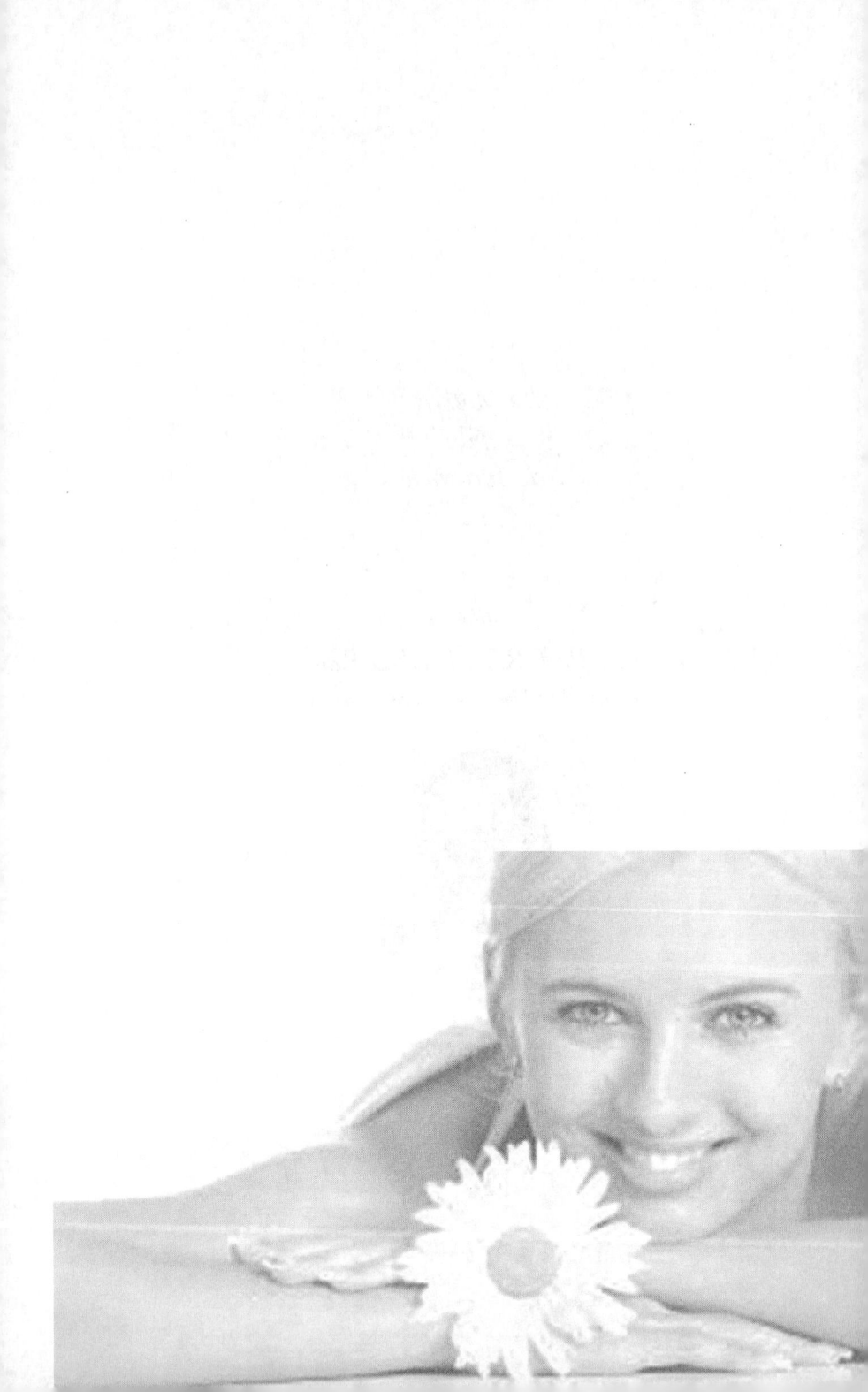

Foreword

It is indeed a great privilege for me to write the Foreword for the book *Textbook of Herbal Cosmetics*, authored by my protégé Prof (Dr) Vimala Devi, former Head, Department of Pharmaceutical Technology. I had been associated with her since 1959 and I had the privilege of observing her keen interest in herbal and phytochemistry. As at that time we were under the umbrella of distinguished Prof S Rangaswamy, a legendary figure who needs no introduction. As such it is indeed laudable that Prof (Dr) Vimala Devi has penned this unique book, keeping in mind that India has a fascinating beauty culture made of traditional natural herbs bestowed with special health benefits and that India has a huge population of approximately 1.2 billion people awaiting access to cosmetics and cleansing products. Due to more and more Indian females becoming economically self-sufficient and professional, about 150 million of customers are now having access to cosmetic products. Not only that, today's males also want to be well groomed and wish to appear handsome. Foreigners are becoming more and more interested in '**Made in India**' herbal cosmetics. India is emerging as one of the most dynamic herbal cosmetic manufacturing country internationally. Thus, this book will be of immense interest not only to the students of pharmacy, cosmetology, and R&D workers but also of cosmetic manufacturers. Manufacturers are investing huge sums of money on R&D to design their products, keeping in mind the ethos of the middle class consumer's psychological orientation towards the beautification properties and usefulness of herbal ingredients which are safe and efficacious. The chapter on baby care products, body care products, hair care products, dental care and oral hygiene products, and also eye care products like kajals would be of tremendous interest to the readers. The Drug and Cosmetics Act, 1940, under Section 3(aaa) has defined cosmetics as any article intended to be rubbed, poured, sprinkled or sprayed on, or introduced into, or otherwise applied to human body or any part thereof for cleansing, beautifying, promoting attractiveness, or altering the appearance and include any article intended for use as component of cosmetics. *Per se* the

Act has not separately defined herbal cosmetics. However, it may be that a cosmetic base whose standard conformed to the schedule of the Drug and Cosmetic Rules, 1945, or as specified by the Bureau of Indian Standards. It would be wise to accept the specification of the herbal component to identify the quality through the marker compound as given for the various herbal components in the Ayurvedic pharmacopeias or Indian pharmacopeia or any other pharmacopeia of a country recognized by Government of India, Ministry of Health, and Ayush on a reciprocating basis. Further cognizance have been taken of traditional knowledge and art and science of manufacture of herbal cosmetics in consonance with international requirement of the content of heavy metals like lead, arsenic, cadmium and mercury. Freedom from untoward side reactions, toxic and allergic manifestations and safety parameters of cosmetics product as laid down by the Bureau of Indian Standards have been taken care of each herb, the pictures of each of cosmetic effective herbs will add a new dimension to the book, which will be of immense help to the readers of this useful book. The book has also taken care while presenting the formulations to built the quality of product during various stages of manufacture and just not tests the final quality of the product; this is the essence of quality assurance. Microbial and oxidative preservation and prevention of oxidative degradation of the formulations are given. I am confident that this book will be a path-breaking original and lucid information resource for anyone interested in herbal cosmetics written by Prof (Dr) Vimala Devi, who has dedicated herself to extensive and intensive original research in this fascinating field of herbal cosmetics. I wish her book all success.

Prof Emeritus BK Gupta
Former Head, Department of Pharmaceutical Technology
Jadavpur University, Kolkata
Acharya PC Ray Memorial Medalist
Andhra University Gold Medalist (1958)
Life Time Achievement Award Winner (2012)
IPA-Ramanbhai Patel Foundation
Chairman, Gluconate-Health Ltd (a Govt. of West Bengal Undertaking)
Director, West Bengal Pharmaceutical and Photochemical Corporation
(a Govt. of West Bengal Undertaking)
Principal Advisor, Emami Ltd, and Member, Zandu Foundation for Health Care

bijangupta@gmail.com

Preface

The concept and importance of herbal cosmetics is ever increasing.

The subject of cosmetics was touched upon only as a small insignificant portion in pharmaceutical technology. Now it is an independent and increasingly important subject in the graduate curriculum.

The term 'herbal cosmetics' is tricky and not defined precisely. The norms on manufacturing and quality control are still in the process of being laid down.

A modest attempt has been made to give a comprehensive information on a few categories of herbal cosmetics.

Baby Care Products

Body Care Products

Hair Care Products

Dental Care and Oral Hygiene Products

M. Vimaladevi

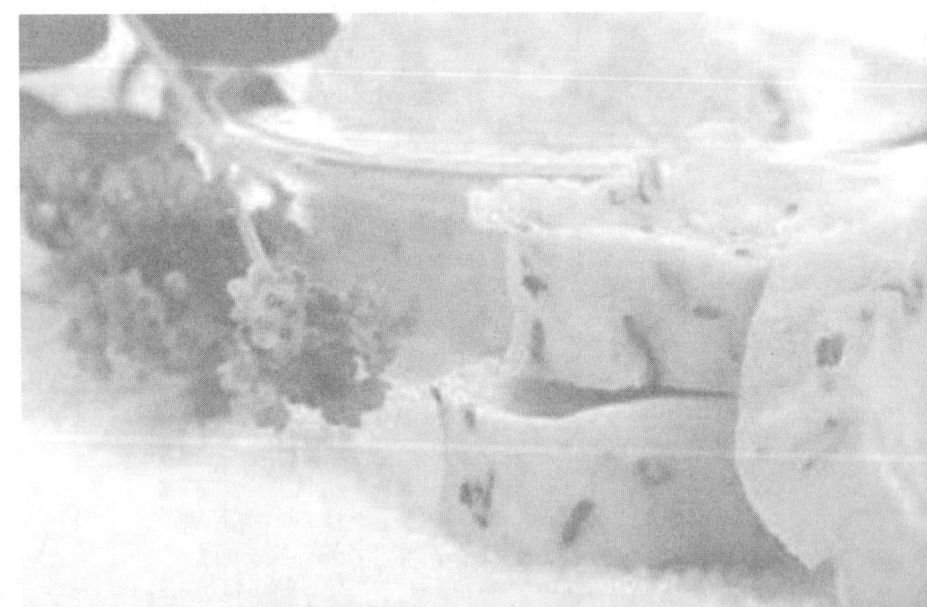

Acknowledgements

I fondly acknowledge the encouragement and help my children have provided me at all stages in the compilation of this volume and thereafter at the time of its production. I greatly admire and cherish their support without which my attempt of writing this book would have remained a distant dream.

I further thank profusely Prof PN Murthy (Berhampur, Odisha), Prof BK Gupta (Kolkata), and Prof CK Kokate (Belgaum), for their invaluable guidance and encouragement.

I am indebted to my manager and PA Mrs UR Vijayalakshmi, for her constant encouragement and assistance.

I also thank my publishers who have transformed my work in the form of a book.

M. Vimaladevi

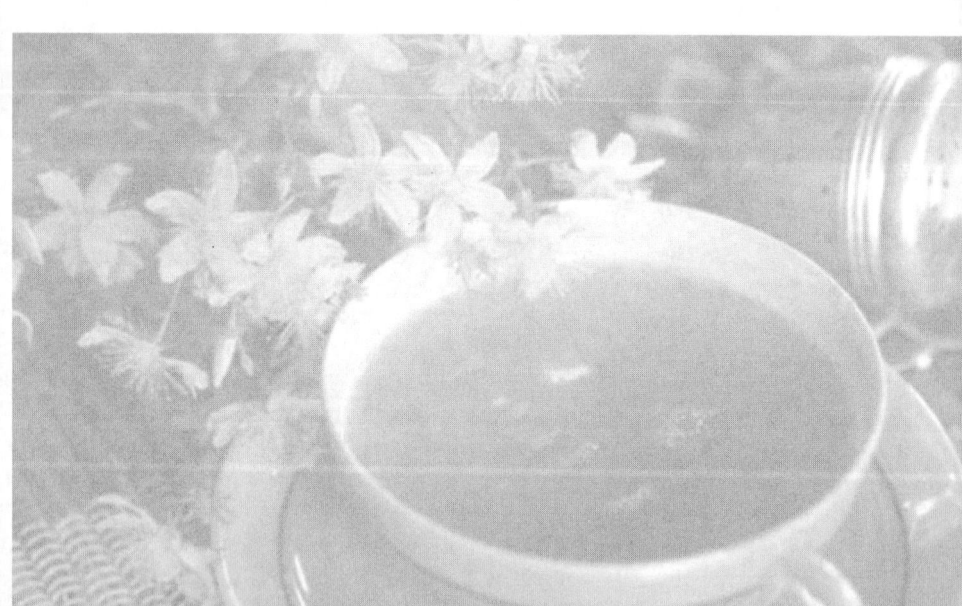

Author's Note

1. Herbal formulations can be assured for quality with the comparison of the raw materials with both green and brown standards. Fresh/green standards are available but not in their dried (brown) form. Since they are not available, quality control and assurance becomes incomplete, unless and until a marker compound, which is responsible for the performance of the product, is identified.

2. Presently each product is being dealt with individually with its respective proprietary standards.

3. Since for each product relevant parameters or instruments are not readily available, the evaluation is mostly qualitative.

4. On cosmetic plant ingredients, neither scientific and systematic manufacturing nor quality control could be dealt comprehensively. It can be done when comprehensive information or monographs of plants or herbs is available. I am hopeful, that this will be made available from our pharmacognosy and phytochemist experts in due course of time. Till such time proprietary standards are to be designed and developed by the manufacturer.

5. Actually the quality control is two dimensional. One is adapting the existing standards of similar products (cosmetics) and wherever it is appropriate and adapting, 2nd dimension is on plants standards, which is already mentioned in my author's note. These two dimensions are to be kept in mind. But it is still in the thought process and can materialise only when plant standards as cosmetic ingredients are declared.

Future Scope for Research—*Suggestions*

1. Development of monographs on the plants useful in herbal cosmetic products for design and development.

2. To develop a few herbal vehicles/bases for the herbal cosmetic products.

3. Screening of plants that can be useful in herbal cosmetic formulations.
4. To identify the marker compound(s) in these plants, which can help in quality control maintenance and sustenance and assurance.

M. Vimaladevi

Contents

Contents

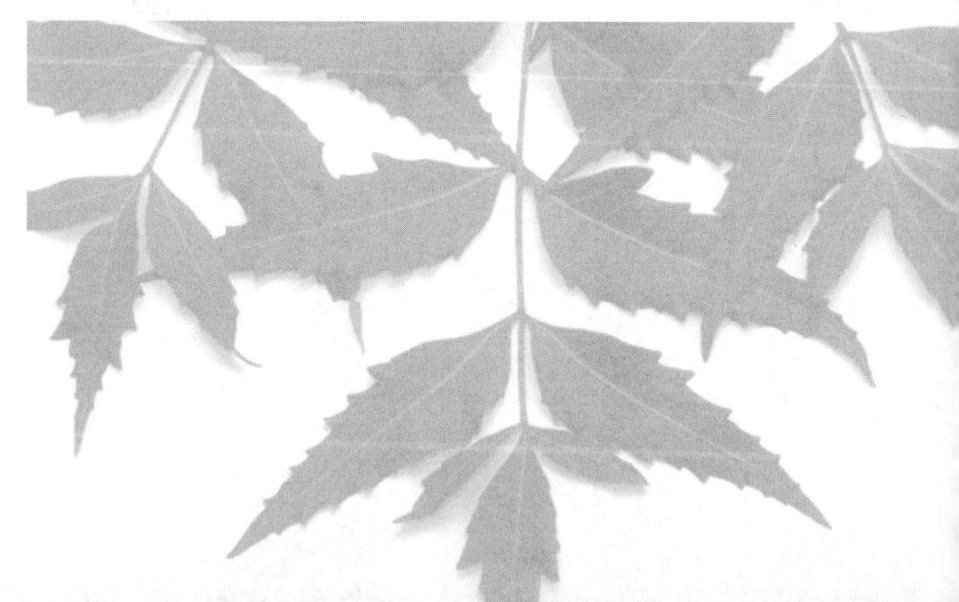

Plate 1

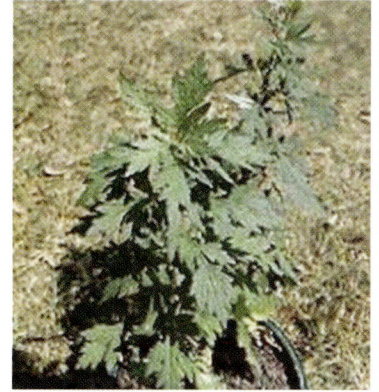

Artemisia vulgaris

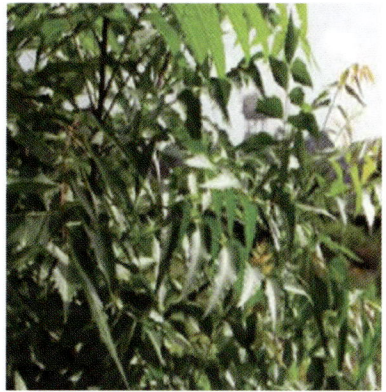

Azadirachta indica

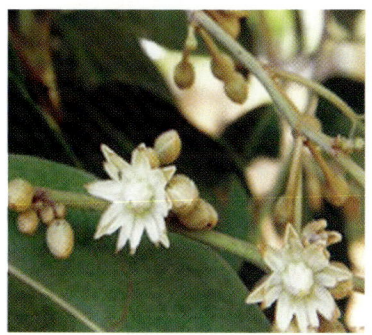

Mimusops elengi

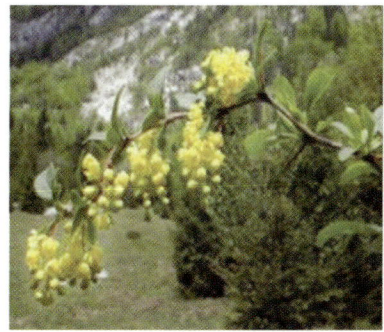

Berberis aristata

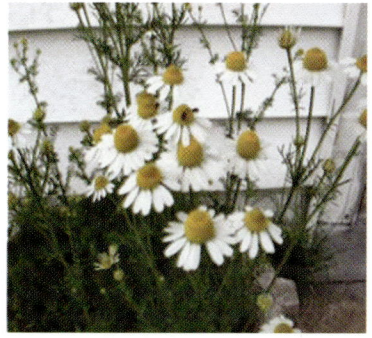

Matricaria chamomilla

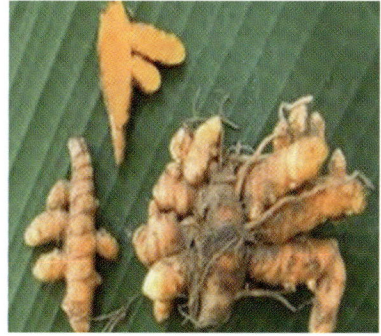

Curcuma aromatica

Plate 2

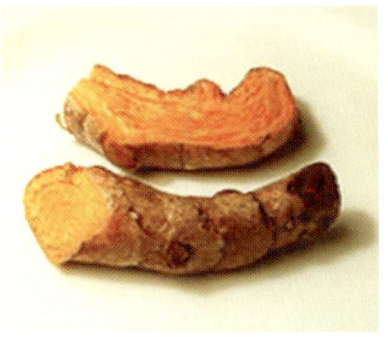

Curcuma longa

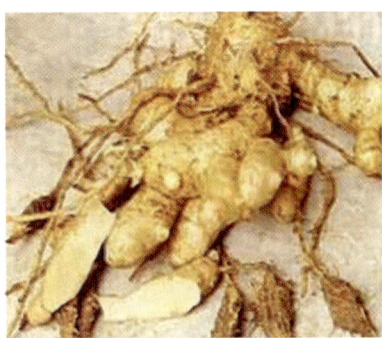

Curcuma zedoaria

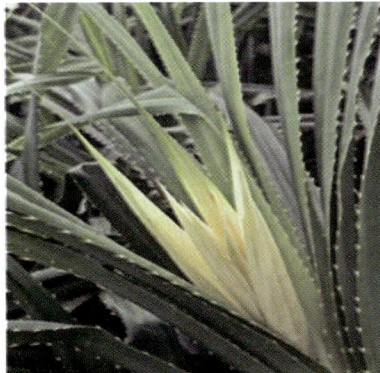

Pandanus odoratissimus

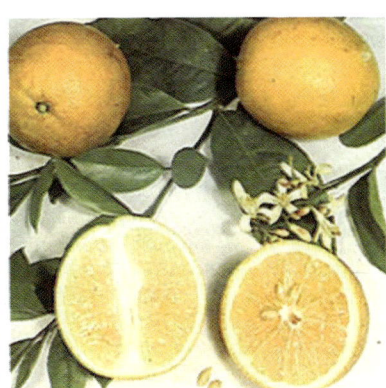

Citrus limon

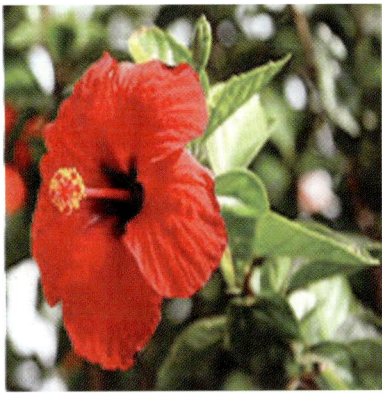

Hibiscus rosa sinensis

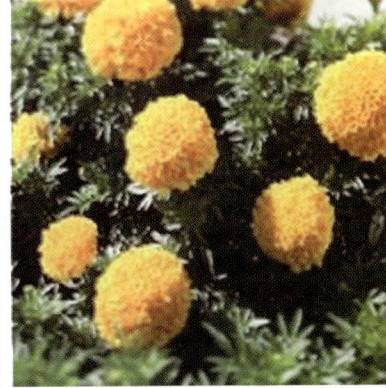

Tagetes erecta

Plate 3

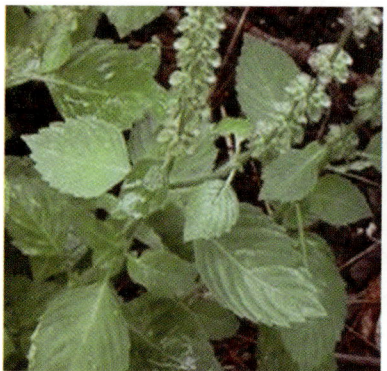

Ocimum sanctum

Citrus aurantious

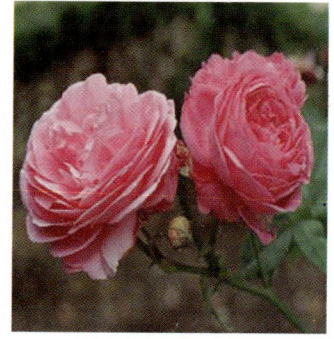

Rosa louise odier

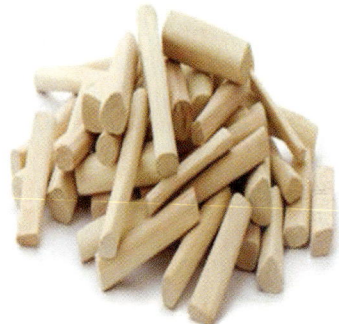

Santalum album

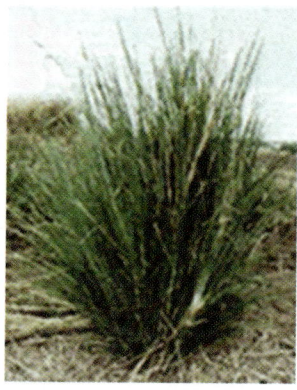

Vetiveria zizanioides

Plate 4

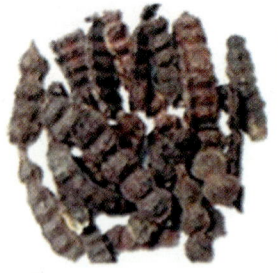
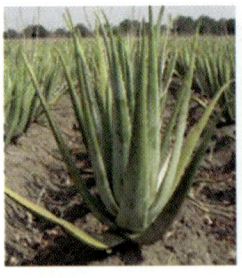
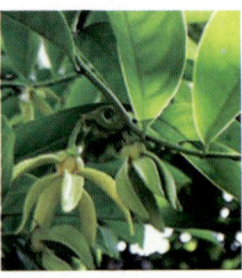

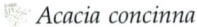
Acacia concinna   *Aloe barbadensis*   *Artabotrys odoratissimus*

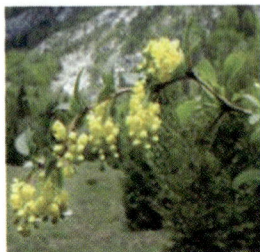
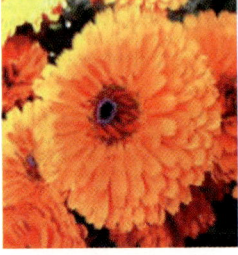

Berberis aristata   *Calendula officinalis*

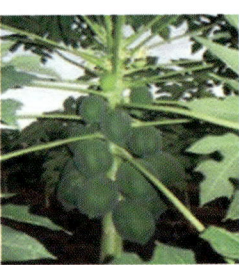
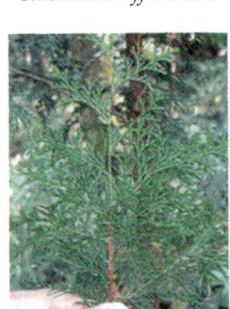

Carica papaya   *Chamecyparia obtusa*

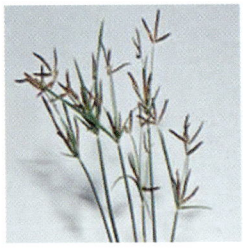
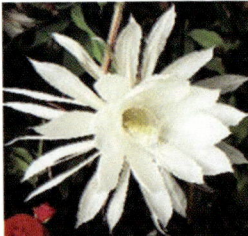

Cyperus rotandus   *Epiphyllum oxypetalum*

Plate 5

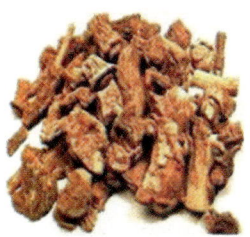
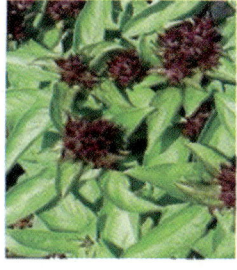
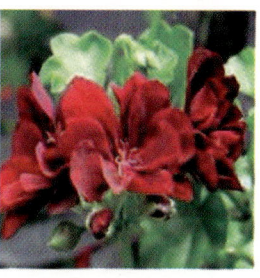

Hemidesmus indicus   *Ocimum basilicum*   *Pelargonium peltatum*

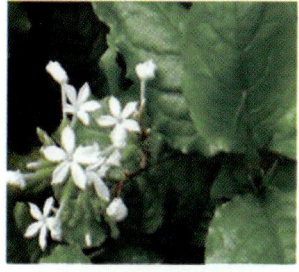
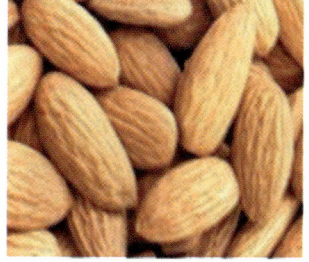

Plumbago indica   *Prunus amygdalus*

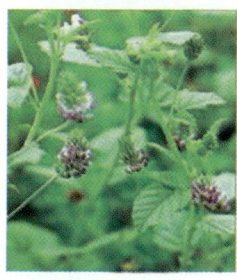
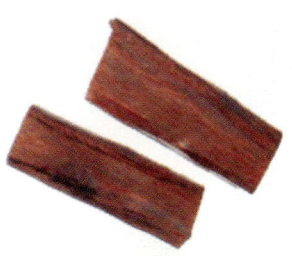

Psoralea cordifolia   *Pterocarpus santalinus*

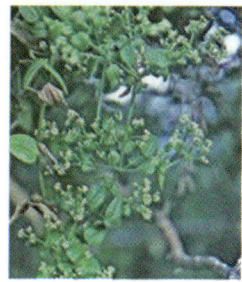
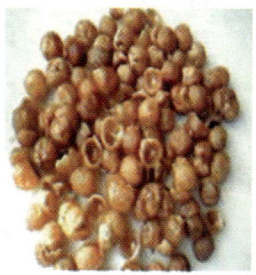

Rubia cordifolia   *Sapindus mukorossi*

Plate 6

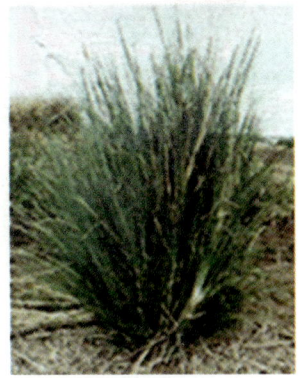

Vetiveria zizanioides

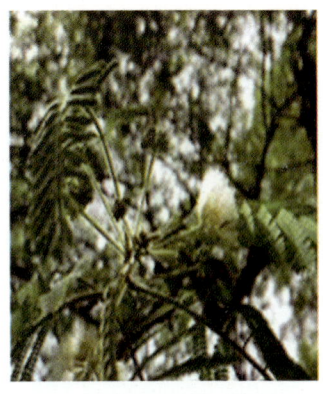

Albizzia amara

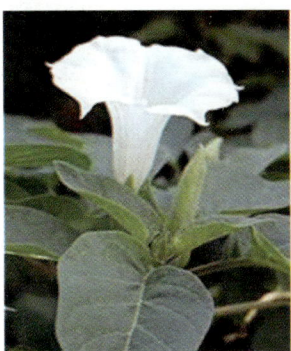

Datura metel

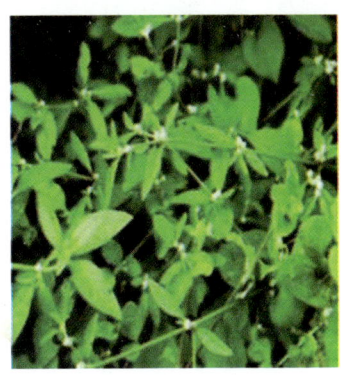

Alternanthera sessilis

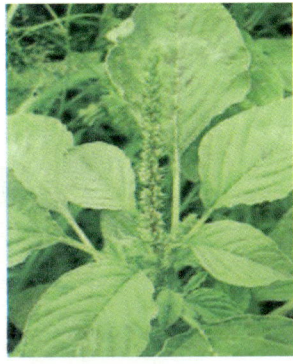

Amaranthus spinosus

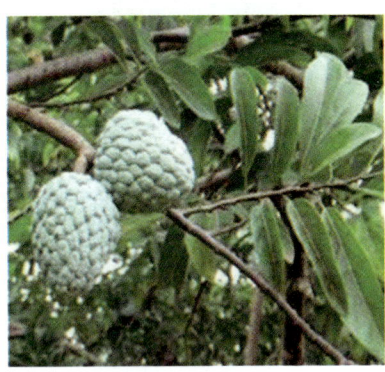

Annona squamosa

Plate 7

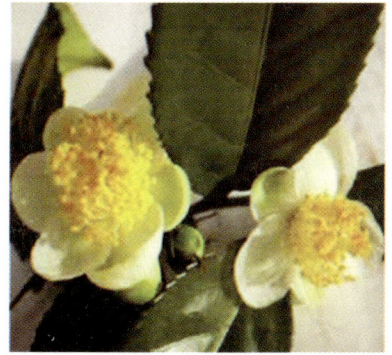

Camellia sinensis

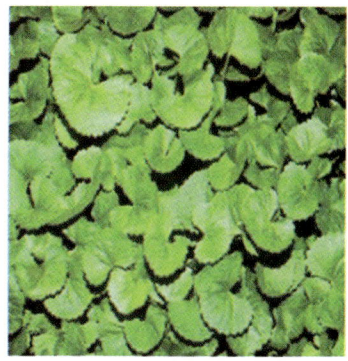

Centella asiatica

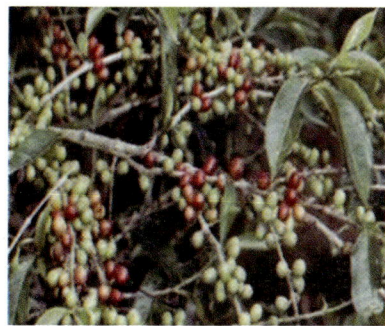

Coffea arabica

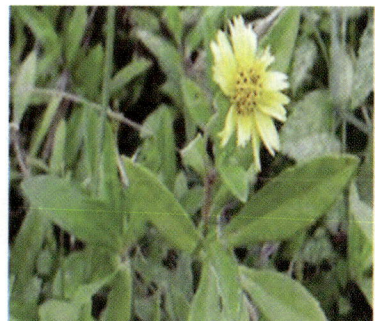

Eclipta alba

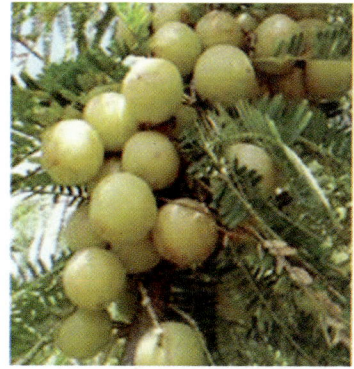

Emblica officinalis

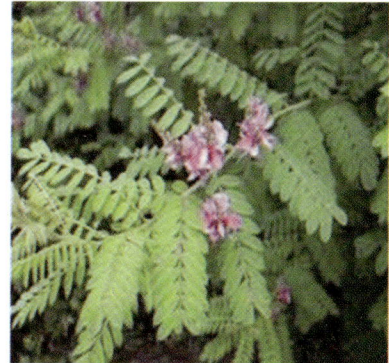

Indigofera tinctoria

Plate 8

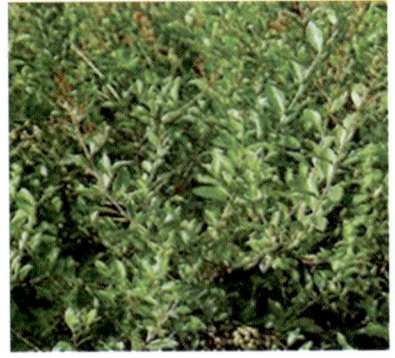

Lawsonia inermis

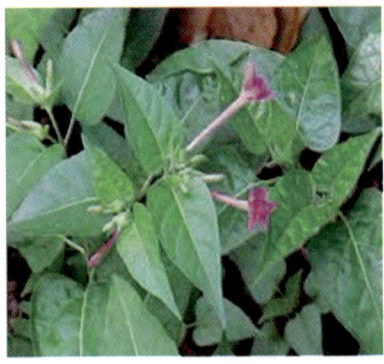

Mirabilis jalapa

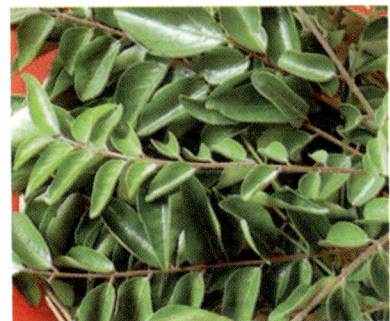

Muraya koenigii

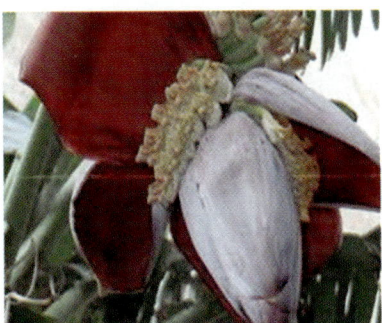

Musa acuminata—flower

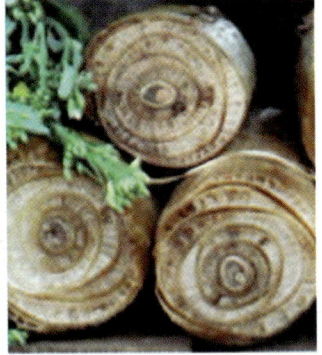

Musa acuminata—root

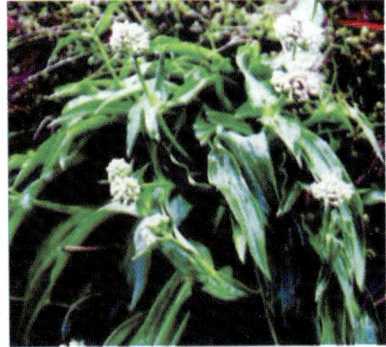

Nardostachys jatamansi

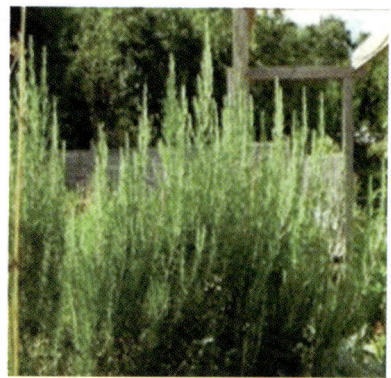

Quercus infectoria

Rosmarinus officinalis

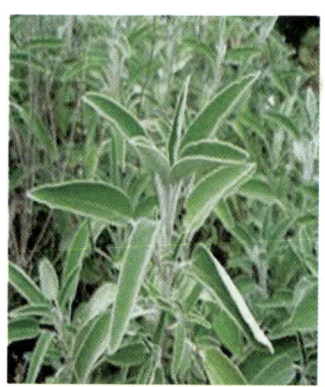

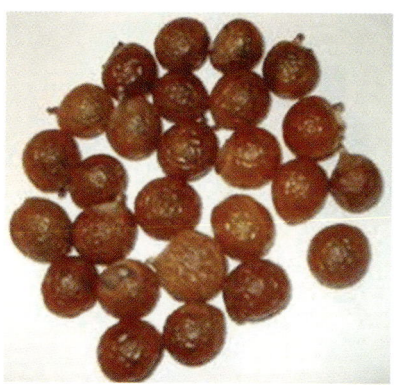

Salvia officinalis

Sapindus mukorossi

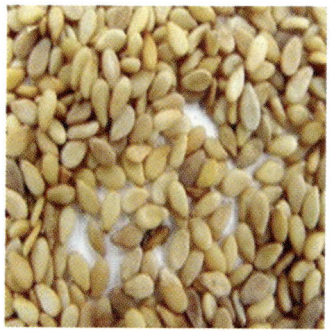

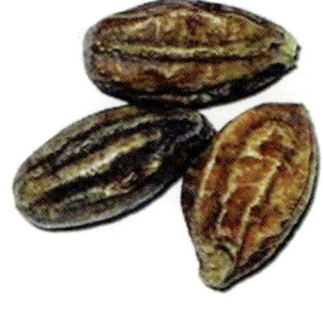

Sesamum indicum

Terminalia chebula

Plate 10

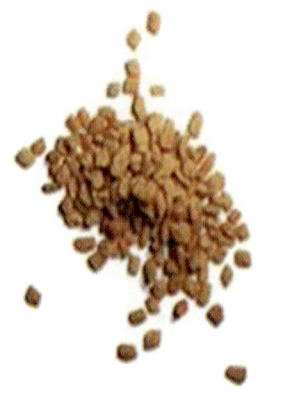

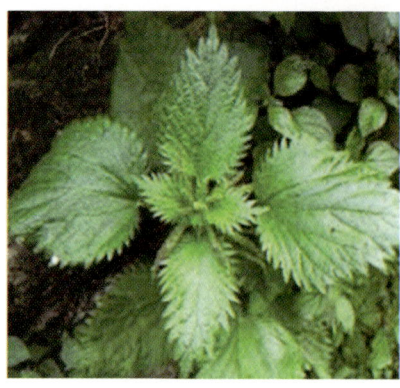

Trigonella foenum-graecum

Urtica dioica

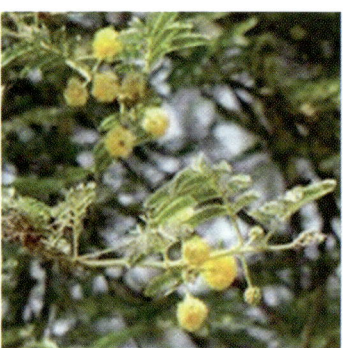

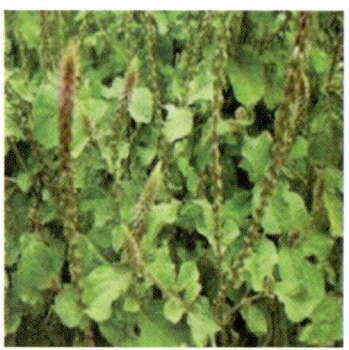

Acacia arabica

Achyranthes aspera

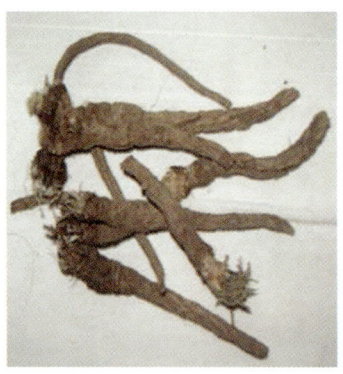

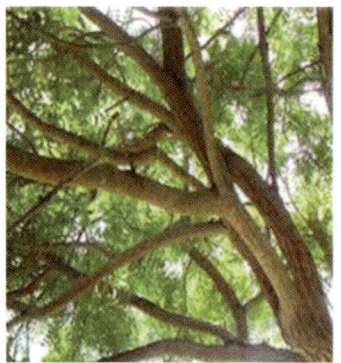

Anacyclus pyrethrum

Azadirachta indica

Plate 11

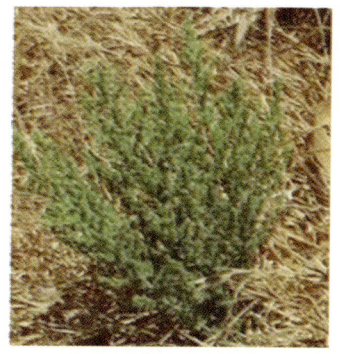

Cressa cretica

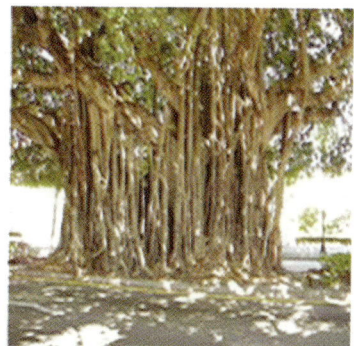

Ficus benghalensis

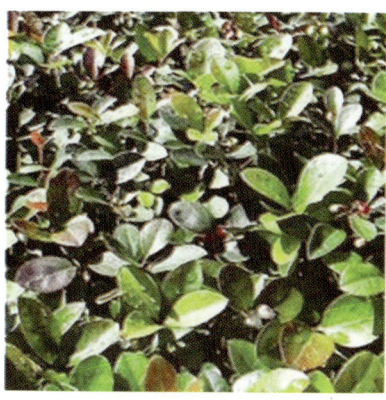

Gaultheria procumbens

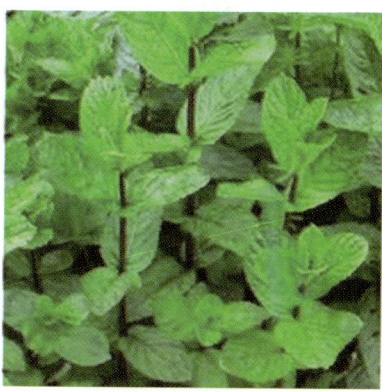

Mentha piperita

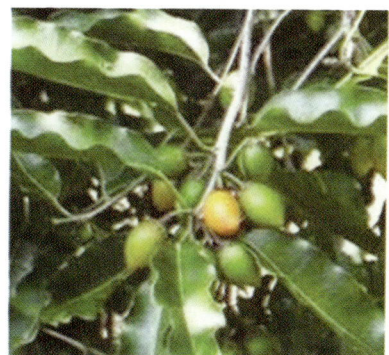

Mimusops elengi

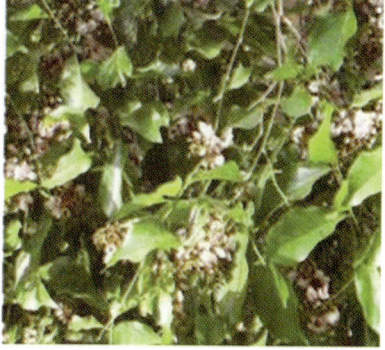

Pongamia glabra

Plate 12

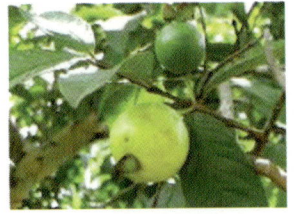

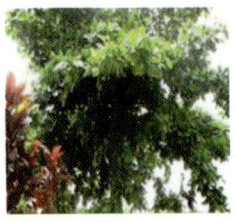

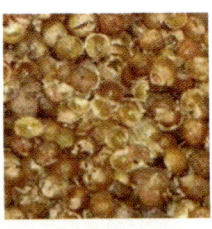

Psidium guajava　　　*Prunus amygdalus*　　　*Sapindus mukorossi*

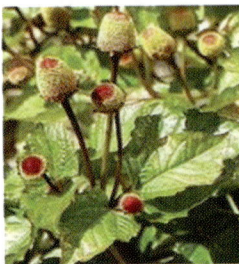

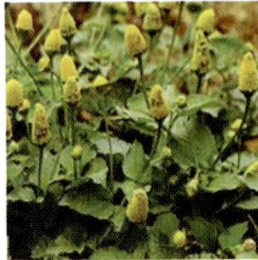

Spilanthes acmella　　　　　　*Spilanthes calva*

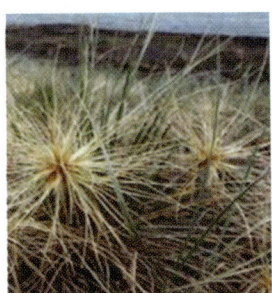

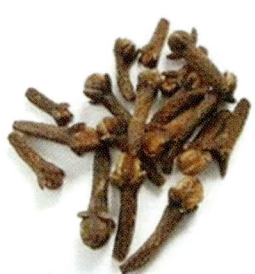

Spinifex squarrosus　　　　　*Syzygium aromaticum*

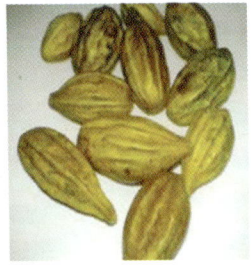

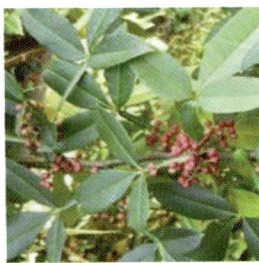

Terminalia chebula　　　　　*Zanthoxylum armatum*

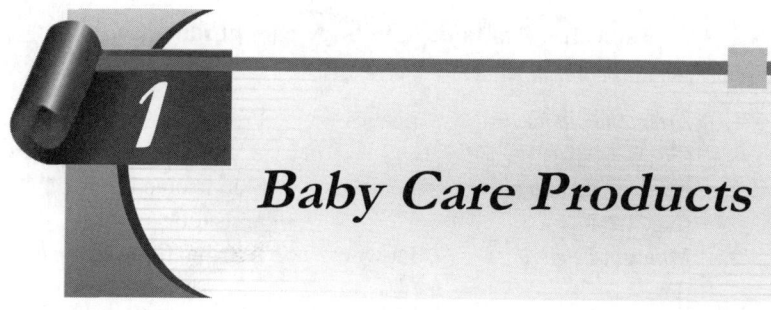

Baby Care Products

Baby toiletries/cosmetics have a special touch to the baby skin, as it is tender, delicate and vulnerable to infections (sometimes), insect bites, etc. Hence, special care and attention are needed in their formulation.

In subcontinental conditions (like in India), babies are given an oil bath twice a day particularly in the warmer months from the day they are born for about a period of 12 months. Body and head are given an oil massage followed by cleansing and washing using naturally scented flour of pulses like Bengal gram and green gram blended with coated herbal powders.

The skin of babies, particularly newborn, is extremely tender so initially for about 12 months it needs protection from insect bites and climatic changes. Further, it needs little massage, for toning up and growth of muscular tissues.

Different categories of baby care products include:

- Massage/bath oils
- Bath powders
- Massage creams
- Body powders
- Shampoos

Table 1.1: Plants used in baby care products

S. No.	Herbs (Botanical name)	Parts used	Property/use
1.	Artemesia vulgaris (Fig. 1.1)	Leaves	Protective/antiseptic
2.	Azadirachta indica (Fig. 1.2)	Leaves	Skin protective, antiseptic
3.	Mimusops elengi (Fig. 1.3)	Flowers	Astringent, fragrance
4.	Berberis aristata (Fig. 1.4)	Roots	Fungicide, antibacterial
5.	Matricaria chamomilla (Fig. 1.5)	Flowers	Relaxant
6.	Curcuma aromatica (Fig. 1.6)	Rhizomes	Protective, antiseptic, fragrance
7.	Curcuma longa (Fig. 1.7)	Rhizomes	Freshening, fragrance, antiseptic
8.	Curcuma zedoaria (Fig. 1.8)	Rhizomes	Fragrance, skin protective
9.	Pandanus odoratissimus (Fig. 1.9)	Flower dust/pollen	Fragrance, refreshing
10.	Citrus limon (Fig. 1.10)	Rinds	Fragrance, refreshing, soothing
11.	Hibiscus rosa sinensis (Fig. 1.11)	Flowers	Conditioning in hair shampoos
12.	Tagetes erecta (Fig. 1.12)	Flowers, leaves	Antiseptic
13.	Ocimum sanctum (Fig. 1.13)	Leaves	Antiseptic, skin protective
14.	Citrus aurantious (Fig. 1.14)	Rinds	Deodorant freshening
15.	Rosa louise odier (Fig. 1.15)	Petals	Astringent, fragrance
16.	Santalum album (Fig. 1.16)	Wood	Protective, complexion improving
17.	Vetiveria zizanioides (Fig. 1.17)	Roots	Refreshing, cooling

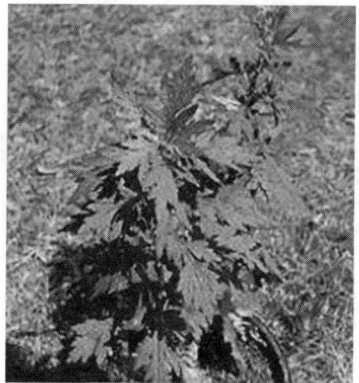

Fig. 1.1: *Artemisia vulgaris*

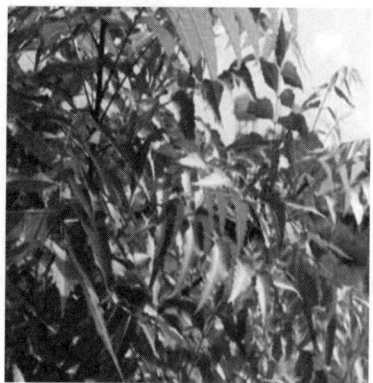

Fig. 1.2: *Azadirachta indica*

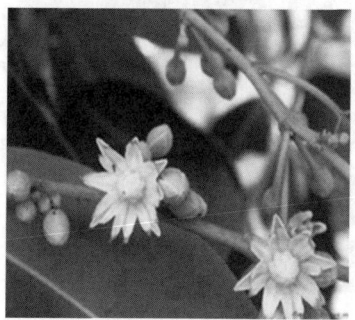

Fig. 1.3: *Mimusops elengi*

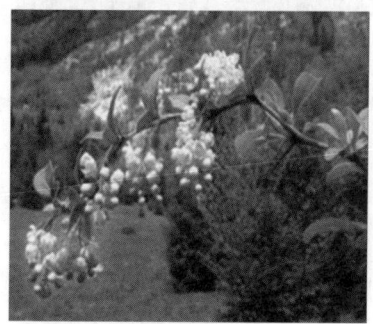

Fig. 1.4: *Berberis aristata*

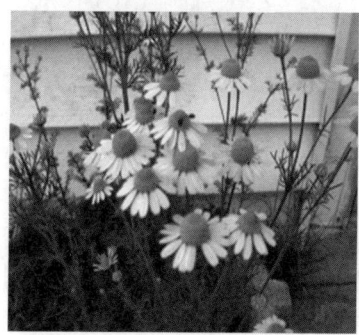

Fig. 1.5: *Matricaria chamomilla*

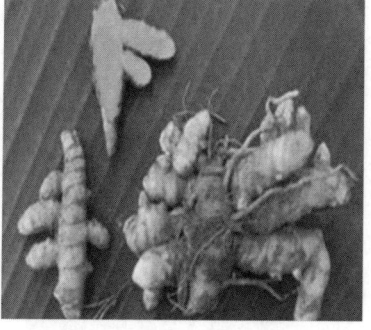

Fig. 1.6: *Curcuma aromatica*

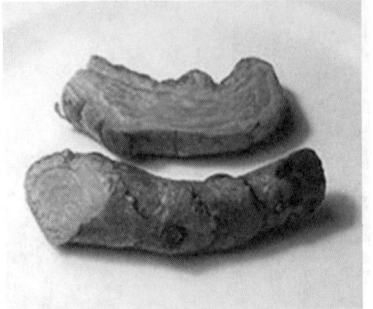

Fig. 1.7: *Curcuma longa*

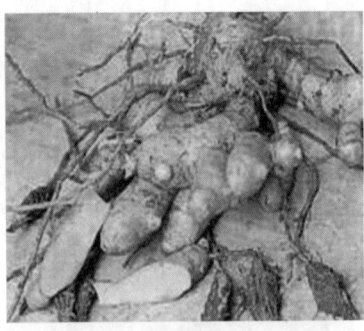

Fig. 1.8: *Curcuma zedoaria*

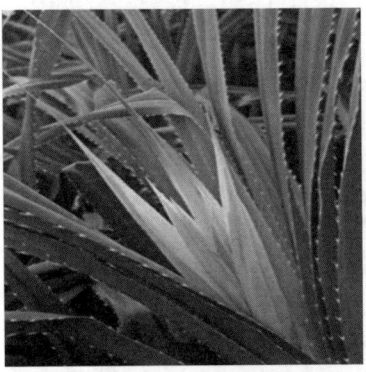

Fig. 1.9: *Pandanus odoratissimus*

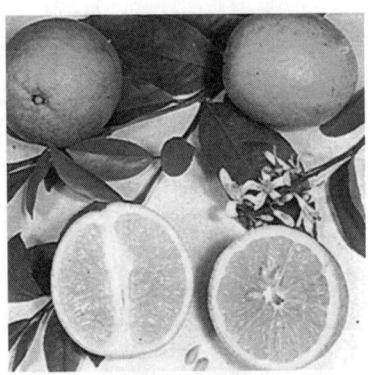

Fig. 1.10: *Citrus limon*

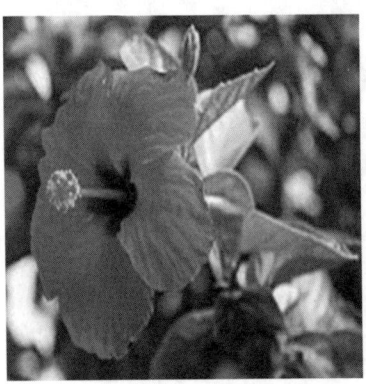

Fig. 1.11: *Hibiscus rosa sinensis*

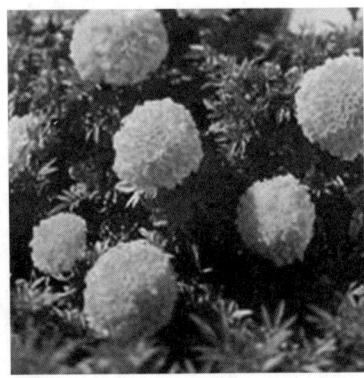

Fig. 1.12: *Tagetes erecta*

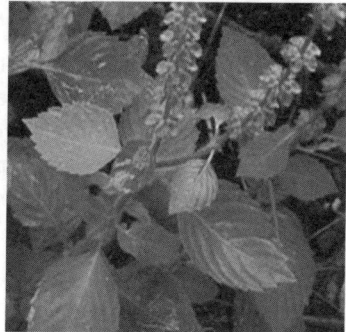

Fig. 1.13: *Ocimum sanctum*

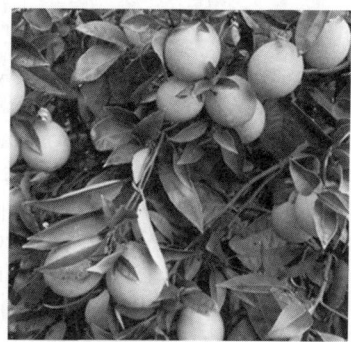

Fig. 1.14: *Citrus aurantious*

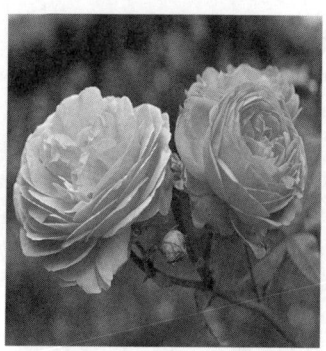

Fig. 1.15: *Rosa louise odier*

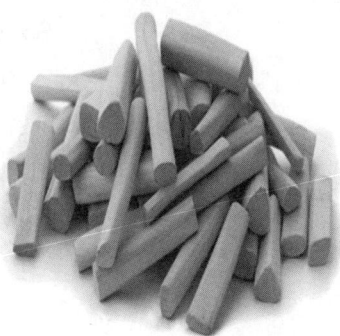

Fig. 1.16: *Santalum album*

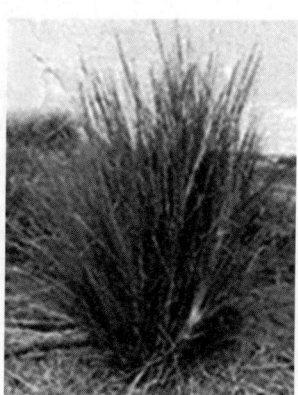

Fig. 1.17: *Vetiveria zizanioides*

BABY MASSAGE OILS

As discussed in the earlier section, in India, babies are given bath twice a day after massaging with baby massage oil followed by cleansing with bath powder. The purpose of using massage oils which are generally vegetable oils like til, mustard, castor, coconut or peanut oil is to help in toning up the muscular tissues of the baby and also to protect its skin from climatic changes.

Here are some useful combinations:
- Gingelly (til) oil and 10% of coconut oil.
- Herbal extract mix
- Deodorised castor oil + coconut oil + turmeric extract. (*see* Tables 1.2 to 1.6).

Formulations

Table 1.2

Base			Herbal extracts		
S. No.	Oil	%	S. No.	Ingredient	Parts
1.	Castor oil	80	1.	Curcuma longa	2
2.	Coconut oil	20	2.	Azadirachta indica	3

Table 1.3

Base			Herbal extracts		
S. No.	Oil	%	S. No.	Ingredient	Parts
1.	Gingelly oil	75	1.	Artemesia vulgaris	3
2.	Peanut oil	20	2.	Ocimum kilim and scharicum	2
3.	Olive oil	5	3.	Mimusops elengi	2
			4.	Vettiveria zizanioides	2

Table 1.4

Base			Herbal extracts		
S. No.	Oil	%	S. No.	Ingredient	Parts
1.	Gingelly oil	80	1.	Berberis aristata	3
2.	Mustard oil	10	2.	Curcuma aromatica	2
3.	Coconut oil	10	3.	Vettiveria zizanioides	1

Table 1.5

Base			Herbal extracts		
S. No.	*Oil*	*%*	*S. No.*	*Ingredient*	*Parts*
1.	Gingelly oil	80	1.	*Azadirachta indica*	3
2.	Peanut oil	10	2.	*Artemesia vulgaris*	2
3.	Castor oil	5	3.	*Berberis aristata*	3
4.	Olive oil	5			

Table 1.6

Base			Herbal extracts mix		
S. No.	*Oil*	*%*	*S. No.*	*Ingredient*	*Parts*
1.	Gingelly (til) oil	80	1.	*Azadirachta indica*	3
2.	Almond oil	5	2.	*Artemesia vulgaris*	3
3.	Rice bran oil	5	3.	*Curcuma longa*	2
4.	Castor oil	2			
5.	Sunflower oil	8			

The absorption of vegetable oils is superior as compared to that of mineral oils. Most of the commercial formulations are blended with synthetic and mineral oils as a result of which the benefits of vegetable oils are reduced.

Usually formulations use sesame oil or olive oil. It may be noted that therapeutically sesame oil and olive oil have more or less similar properties. Coconut oil is not used in these formulations as it has a tendency to attract ants.

In India, vegetable oils are a popular choice. However, olive oil has caught the attention of most Indian mothers because of the hype. It is not of Indian origin but imported from Spain or Italy. As this oil is not indigenous, there is an ample scope for adulteration with other oils particularly in repackaged packs. As already discussed, sesame oil may not have the glamour of olive oil, but therapeutically they have similar qualities with respect to toning of the skin and nutritional value (skin food). Castor oil is used more for its protective application, for protecting and preventing from any insect bite. Due to its high viscosity, insects find it difficult to crawl on the body.

Baby massage oils are meant for massaging the body of the baby a few minutes before the baby bath. 5% mustard oil can be added to the base sesame oil as it is heat generating. Massage helps in improving blood circulation and maintenance of stature structure and shining of skin.

Manufacturing

The vegetable oils mixed with the herbal extracts are put together and slowly heated at 70°C, till the extract is transferred to the oil phase. Then it is decanted slowly and dried till the oil is free from moisture. Moisture may lead to rancidity which is undesirable. Hence, the dried or moisture free oil is stored in a cool place. A slow process of manufacturing is keeping it in sun for 2 weeks. The base is a blend of vegetable oils preferably sesame oil and mustard oil as both of them have good toning effect on the muscles, particularly tender muscles. These are nourishing to the skin as well. The addition of certain herbs like *Curcuma longa*, *Artemesia vulgaris* and *Curcuma aromatica* help provide an antiseptic effect on the skin and others like *Vetiveria zizanioides*, *Hemidesmus indicus* to give the skin a glowy, smooth texture, fragrance and freshness.

Direction to Use

The baby oils are generally applied to the entire body of the baby with a gentle massage before bath for ten minutes till the oil is completely absorbed by the skin which can be taken as end point and the baby is kept in the sun (sunbathe) for 10 minutes. Then the residual oily film if any on the baby skin is cleansed with bath powder containing either Bengal gram or herbal bath powder consisting of green gram, moong dal or whole moong with powdered herbs mixed in it.

Baby Bath Oils

The baby massage oils, enriched with herbal extracts like *Artemesia vulgaris*, *Curcuma aromatica*, *Vetiveria zizanioides* will not only protect the tender skin of the baby but also give it a pleasant odour and keep it fresh for long hours.

Baby Massage Oils

The oleo extracts of plants or plant parts that are useful in herbal baby oil include *Arazadirachta indica, Berberis aristata* and *Mimusops elengi* flowers or floral extracts of flowers or floral extracts. It is a common practice to soak parts of an aromatic plant either leaves, roots or bark in the vegetable oil such that some constituents of the essential oil of the plant get dissolved in the oil and a natural fragrance is imparted to the oil, e.g. *Michalea champa, Mimusops elengi* flowers.

Traditionally, in India, powders of the herbs are mixed in the base oil and set aside till a portion of the essential oil of the plant is extracted by the base oil. Then the oil would be decanted and used and stored, when it is moisture free.

As mentioned earlier, vegetable oils have an edge over synthetic substituents like IPM or silicones, as far as absorption is concerned whereas the latter are less greasy than the vegetable oils. However, if the absorption advantage is to be considered, vegetable oils are preferred. But the vegetable oils have disadvantage of a shorter shelf life as they tend to turn rancid. The formulator has to use his/her expertise in blending the raw materials, the vegetable oils and synthetic oils or along with antioxidants in a judicious proportion taking into account both advantages and disadvantages in providing an ideal product to the consumer.

Manufacturing

The herbal extracts and oil base is heated for four hours at 50°C, or kept in sun for two weeks, till the oil is free from any moisture.

Quality Control

Oil should be free from moisture, transparent and yellowish green in colour. Colour, refractive index, specific gravity, and viscosity are to be checked.

Packing and Storage

Packed in unit packs of 100 or 200 ml in glass bottles with air tight lids and stored away from light and heat. Bulk oil is stored in stainless steel (ss) tanks.

Evaluation

The oil should be absorbed by the skin and spreadable (lubricant), i.e. 5 ml over 10 sq.cm. in 5 min. Good absorption, penetrability, lubrication and spreadability are to be evaluated.

BABY BATH POWDERS

After the massage of baby's skin with baby massage oil, it is an age-old practice in India to apply a naturally scented bath powder using flour of pulses as base blended with *Curcuma longa, Curcuma zedoaria, Vetiveria zizanioides* and *Santalum album* to cleanse the body of the baby. This helps in keeping it free from skin affections, infections and fresh with fragrance of the above mentioned scented powders. Once a week, the general baby bath powder fortified with the addition of a herbal powder mix may be used for better results.

Formulations

Table 1.7

Base			Herbal powder mix		
S. No.	Ingredient	%	S. No.	Ingredient	Parts
1.	Pulse powder	80	1.	Artemesia vulgaris	3
2.	Green gram: Bengal gram (80:20)	10	2.	Majona leaf	2
			3.	Cyprus rotandus	3
3.	Mineral—Multani mitti Herbal powder mix	10	4.	Curcuma aromatica	4

Table 1.8

Base			Herbal powder mix		
S. No.	Ingredient	%	S. No.	Ingredient	Parts
1.	Bengal gram flour	50	1.	Azadirachta indica	5
2.	Green gram flour	30	2.	Santalum album	5
3.	Rice flour	5	3.	Curcuma zedoaria	5
4.	Multani mitti	5	4.	Curcuma aromatica	5
5.	Herbal powder mix	10	5.	Vetiveria zizanioides	5

A mixture of all these herbs is finely powdered, sieved through 80 mesh and mixed in one of the base pulse powders. It can be used for cleaning oily skin as well as the head of the babies previously massaged with baby oils.

Some babies and children are allergic to moong dal and so it can be substituted by Bengal gram or horse gram.

Note: Baby bath powder can be made with whole moong powder instead of moong dal powder for children up to one year. Herbal bath powder can be used for the head and body.

Manufacturing

The base powder and herbal mix powder are thoroughly mixed in a double cone blender.

All the above mentioned herbal parts are thoroughly shade dried and powdered and sieved through 100 mesh, to remove any fibrous material and little camphor is added for the purpose of preservation and also to prevent the tender skin of the baby from insect bite.

Quality Control

The powder should freely pass through a 100 mesh sieve.

Packing and Storage

Unit doses are filled in a polyethylene bag, sealed and packed in an outer carton.

Evaluation

After bathing with this powder, the skin of the baby should be free from grease and any residual dirt, fresh and fragrant.

BABY CREAMS

Creams are in general semisolid external preparations, prepared out of oil, water and emulsifiers. Creams can be recommended as substitute for oils, as the absorption and penetration is easier and faster than those of the oils with a pleasant feel on the skin. In addition, creams have another advantage: They can be applied after giving the baby a bath and as a result it remains on the skin for a longer period of time unlike the baby bath oils most of which are washed away.

Among the vegetable oils used as bases for creams, almond oil is the most preferred followed by olive oil and thirdly a mixture of the two oils in varying proportion. These are nutritive creams with a cosmetic appeal.

The baby herbal creams are both oil in water—o/w (massage) and water in oil—w/o (cleansing) emulsions.

a. O/w creams are hydrophilic and leave a thin film of protective nature on the skin. Due to rapid evaporation of water from the rich water content cream, it gives a cooling effect.

b. W/o type of creams, leave a hydrophobic film (less permeable) on the skin. The evaporation of water from the internal phase is relatively slow and is preferable for babies.

The antiseptic activity is imparted to the baby herbal creams, with *Azadirachta* leaf and *Curcuma longa* extracts, along with *Artemesia vulgaris* leaf extract, which acts as an additional antiseptic to *Azadirachta indica* and *Curcuma longa*.

As protective ingredients, the herbal extracts in use are *Azadirachta indica* leaf, *Artemesia vulgaris* leaf, *Vetiveria zizanioides, Curcuma aromatica* and *Santalum album* oil.

Other vegetable oils or fixed oils that can be selected for making baby creams are til oil, sunflower oil, peanut oil, almond oil and apricot oil.

General formula of a baby cream is given below:

Table 1.9

S. No.	Ingredient	%
1.	Almond oil	80
2.	Apricot oil	16
3.	Til oil	4
4.	Perfume	QS

O/w type of creams contain vegetable oil or oils mix in oily phase (70% and 2% wool fat) and a natural emulsifier like beeswax and borax.

An ideal o/w cream should serve the purpose of softening the baby skin. Good spreadability and ease of application are the important requirements for such creams.

BABY MASSAGE CREAMS

Formulations

Table 1.10

Base			Herbal extracts mix		
S. No.	Ingredient	%	S. No.	Ingredient	Parts
1.	Herbal massage oil	50	1.	Azadirachta indica	10
2.	Beeswax	3	2.	Artemisia vulgaris	5
3.	Borax	2	3.	Tegetes erecta	5
4.	Triethanolamine	5			
5.	Water	40			
6.	Preservatives	QS			
7.	Perfume	QS			

Table 1.11

Base			Herbal extracts mix		
S. No.	Ingredient	%	S. No.	Ingredient	Parts
1.	Olive oil	40	1.	Artemesia vulgaris	2
2.	Beeswax	5	2.	Azadirachta indica	2
3.	Borax	3	3.	Santalum album oil	1
4.	Triethanolamine	4			
5.	Water	32			
6.	Herbal extract mix	6			
7.	Perfume	QS			
8.	Preservatives	QS			

The selection of vegetable oils is the main criterion in preparing the base of w/o creams which are nourishing for the skin. These creams can be used as skin foods or tonics especially for the baby, as they help in the growth of the muscles and skin of the newborn.

Herbal Extracts Used in Creams

Care must be taken to see that the herbal extracts used in the cream should mix uniformly and do not settle down or creep to surface to form a thin layer on the top on standing. It involves skill and expertise in the formulation and manufacture of herbal creams.

It may be noted that it is easier to deal with w/o creams rather than o/w creams. The associated problems include:

1. Rancidity on storage due to high percentage of vegetable oils, which contain lot of unsaturated fatty acids.
2. Because of the difference in densities of herbal extract and the base, there is a likelihood of separation or bleeding of extracts. Hence, care should be taken to avoid this.
3. Instability in the emulsion base due to rich oil content — mostly separation of oil is observed if the percentage and proper ratio of the strong emulgent is not selected.

Preformulation studies should be carried out in these lines before production is taken up on a large scale.

Categories: Baby creams should mostly be

1. Protective
2. Nourishing
3. Muscle toning.

Hence, the selection of base ingredients, followed by herbal extract, is the most critical factor in the baby cream formulations.

BABY MASSAGE CREAMS

The baby massage creams are generally made out of vegetable oils, e.g. olive, sesame, coconut or almond oils. This type of a cream is o/w. Herbal massage creams are more desirable due to the additional properties of the herbs in the cream. In one way, these herbal creams can be called enriched massage creams. As a base, vegetable oils are always desirable due to their beneficial properties. These creams have the advantage as they can be applied to the skin after bath.

A simple way of preparing cosmetic creams for babies or adults is to prepare an o/w type wherein the oily phase is mineral oil. The absorption of mineral oil based cream is relatively less than that of vegetable oil based cream resulting in decreased absorption. Most of the commercial creams are made out of mineral oils and their substitutes like IPM (isopropyl myrstate), silicones, etc. Therefore, a judicious blend of vegetable oils is recommended in the oil phase in creams.

Baby Cream Base

Vegetable oils like almond oil, olive oil, coconut oil, gingelly oil, ricebran oil or mixture of these vegetable oils, can also be taken as an oil phase in making baby massage creams for the tender skin. However, these vegetable oils can turn rancid quickly and their shelf life can be a problem. It can be partly corrected with the addition of a good antioxidant. Looking at the advantages and benefits of vegetable oils, the importance of oil massage to babies as a traditional procedure in India, for the care of tender baby skin can be recalled here. The creams made out of these vegetable oils have a lubricating as well as softening effect on the skin.

O/W Type of Creams

Table 1.12

Base			Herbal extracts mix		
S. No.	Ingredient	%	S. No.	Ingredient	Parts
1.	Vegetable oil—olive oil	50	1.	Matricaria chamomilla	2
2.	Wool fat	3	2.	Curcuma longa	3
3.	Beeswax	4			
4.	Borax	7			
5.	Water	30			
6.	Herbal extract	4			
7.	Antioxidants	2			
8.	Preservatives	QS			
9.	Perfume	QS			

Table 1.13

Base			Herbal extracts mix		
S. No.	Ingredient	%	S. No.	Ingredient	Parts
1.	Vegetable oil—Til oil	45	1.	Tagetes erecta	2
2.	Wool fat	2	2.	Curcuma aromatica	3
3.	Polyglycol monostearate	8			
4.	Spermaceti	5			
5.	Glycol monostearate	5			
6.	Water	30			
7.	Herbal extract	5			
8.	Preservatives	QS			
9.	Perfume	QS			

W/O Type of Creams

Table 1.14

Base			Herbal extracts mix		
S. No.	Ingredient	%	S. No.	Ingredient	Parts
1.	Vegetable oil—apricot oil	30	1.	Curcuma longa	2
2.	Beeswax	3	2.	Artemesia vulgaris	3
3.	Emulsifying wax	2			
4.	Water	60			
5.	Herbal extract	5			
6.	Preservatives	QS			
7.	Perfume	QS			

Manufacturing

Both the phases (oily and aqueous) are heated to 70°C and stirred in a mixing vessel for 15 minutes, then transferred to a colloid mill and when it congeals to a solid mass, it is emptied into a SS storage tank.

Quality Control

Cream should be smooth, soft, non-gritty and lustrous.

Packing and Storage

Packaged in plastic containers or tubes and stored in a cool dry place.

Evaluation

When applied on the skin say 5 g, it should be absorbed over 10 sq.cm. of skin after gentle (o/w type) massage for 5 minutes. The cream should leave a thin film of oily phase or non-greasy, skin should get lustrous, smooth, soft and fragrant.

For cleansing (w/o) cream, covering should not occlude the pores of the skin. It should be smooth, soft, silky, non-gritty, thus leaving mat like film after applying on the skin.

BABY HERBAL POWDERS (BODY AND FACE)

Baby skin is very tender, delicate and vulnerable to infections or any abrasions. The skin has to be protected from any unwanted affections and infections. The folds of tender skin are likely to contract arterial infections. Hence, it is advisable to cover the vulnerable parts with a lubricant powder, preferably of an antiseptic or protective nature. The herbs generally used are *Curcuma longa, Curcuma aromatica, Santalum album, Artemisia vulgaris* leaves, *Azadirachta indica* leaves, *Ocimum sanctum* leaves and camphor.

Special Precautions

It is hard to obtain a fine herbal powder mix because of the different texture each individual powder rhizome brings with it. The second difficulty is in the mixing or blending; there will be a tendency of non-uniformity in blending. However, care must be taken in phases of processing technology to maintain the quality control and assurance.

In the third phase, the problem is in the selection and blending of the perfume. The compatibility of the perfume with the inherent fragrance of the herbal powders mix used as ingredients in the formulation is important. Some examples are scented turmeric, sandal wood, curcuma, zodiac, etc. have their own natural fragrance, the blending within the

a. (intra) ingredients

b. (inter) with perfume, should be carefully and rationally thought of before final the composition. Here is where, the expertise of the perfumer and the formulator is critical.

Strictly speaking an additional perfume is not necessary, as the herbal ingredients themselves have a naturally pleasing fragrance. But for consumer acceptance, it has become imperative to add the perfume occasionally over and above the natural fragrance.

Formulations

Table 1.15

Base			Herbal powder mix		
S. No.	Ingredient	%	S. No.	Ingredient	Parts
1.	Rice starch	30	1.	Santalum album	3
2.	Precipitated chalk	30	2.	Mimusops elengi	2
3.	Light magnesium carbonate	5	3.	Artemesia vulgaris	1
			4.	Azadirachta indica	2
4.	Corn starch	20	5.	Curcuma aromatica	2
5.	Colloidal clay	5			
6.	Herbal powder mix	10			

Table 1.16

Base			Herbal powder mix		
S. No.	Ingredient	%	S. No.	Ingredient	Parts
1.	Talc	70	1.	Vetiveria zizanioides	3
2.	Rice starch	15	2.	Jasminium grandiflorum	2
3.	Magnesium carbonate	5			
4.	Zinc stearate	3			
5.	Magnesium stearate	2			
6.	Herbal powder mix	5			

Table 1.17

Base			Herbal powder mix		
S. No.	Ingredient	%	S. No.	Ingredient	Parts
1.	Talc	70	1.	Azadirachta indica	2
2.	Rice starch	5	2.	Curcuma aromatica	3
3.	Magnesium carbonate	5	3.	Artemesia vulgaris	5
4.	Zinc carbonate	5			
5.	Zinc stearate	3			
6.	Magnesium stearate	2			
7.	Colloidal clay	5			
8.	Herbal powder mix	5			

Manufacturing

All the herbal ingredients are powdered and passed through a 120-mesh and rolled in a triple roller mill once and this mix is blended with the base finally. The blending is carried out in a double cone blender. Preferably leaves and flowers like soft tissue materials are mixed separately. Roots and rhizomes, woody materials like sandalwood are put together and separately powdered.

Quality Control

Quality is checked for adherence and covering. Perfume stability and degree of fragrance is also noted. The fragrance should remain same throughout the shelf life.

Degree of fineness desired: For face—120 mesh screened powder, and for body—80 mesh screened powder.

Packing and Storage

The blended powders are passed through sieve no 80, packed and put into plastic or tin outer containers.

Evaluation

The powder should adhere to the surface of the skin and spread uniformly to protect the skin.

SHAMPOOS

Definition

Shampoos are hair washing or cleansing products with either natural cleansing materials and base or mild surfactants.

Herbal Shampoos

These are hair cleansing products containing herbal ingredients either, the base or in the cleansing phase. Generally the cleansing is done by surfactants or soaps.

Baby Shampoos

Baby's ocular tissue is more sensitive than the adults and hence much care is needed in designing and developing the formulation. The pH should be maintained at 7 such that there is no irritation to the eyes.

Formulations

Table 1.18

Base			Herbal extracts mix		
S. No.	Ingredient	%	S. No.	Ingredient	Parts
1.	Mild surfactant SLES	45	1.	Acacia concinna	3
2.	Cocoamidopropyl betaine	12	2.	Albizzia amara	2
3.	Polyethylene glycol	32			
4.	Distearate	6			
5.	Herbal extract mix	5			
6.	Colour	QS			
7.	Perfume	QS			
8.	Preservatives	QS			

Manufacturing

The ingredients (from base) 1, 2, 3, 4, and 8 are separately mixed and both are added together to give a uniform mixture.

Tearless Baby Shampoo

Table 1.19

Base			Herbal extracts mix		
S. No.	Ingredient	%	S. No.	Ingredient	Parts
1.	Tearless surfactant	40	1.	Acacia concinna	3
2.	Na laureth-2 sulfate	5	2.	Albizzia amara	5
3.	Propylene glycol	3	3.	Hibiscus rosa sinensis	2
4.	Water	46			
5.	Herbal mix	5			
6.	Lauramide DEA	2			

Manufacturing

1. Example: Amphoteric-10, Miranol H2M conc., Miranol Chemical, Irvington, N.J. or Schercopol OMIS–Na, Disodium oleo iso-propanolamide sulfosuccinate, Clifton, N.J.

2. Standapol ES–2, 30% active

3. Superamide L 9, Onyx

Mix in the order shown. Heat to 50°C to dissolve lauramide. pH should be 7.0.

Mild Baby Shampoo

Table 1.20

Base			Herbal extracts mix		
S. No.	Ingredient	%	S. No.	Ingredient	Parts
1.	Sodium lauryl ether sulphate	6	1.	Albizzia amara	3
2.	Cocamidopropyl betaine	12	2.	Acacia concinna	2
3.	Polyoxyethylene sorbitan monolaurate	6			
4.	Polyethylene glycol distearate	1			
5.	Water	70			
6.	Herbal extract mix	5			
7.	Perfume	QS			
8.	Preservatives	QS			

Manufacturing

Mix the ingredients in the order and heat to 70°C and lastly perfume, preservatives, and colour are added and stirred for 15 minutes, allowed to stand overnight and transferred to SS storage tanks for filling.

Quality Control

1. Foam height
2. Stability of foam
3. Viscosity—80 cps
4. pH—7

Packing and Storage

Packed in clear pet bottles or PVC stand-up tubes.

Evaluation

Cleansing, irritation free to eyes and scalp, foam quality, stability, satisfactory miscibility with water, cloud point, hair manageability.

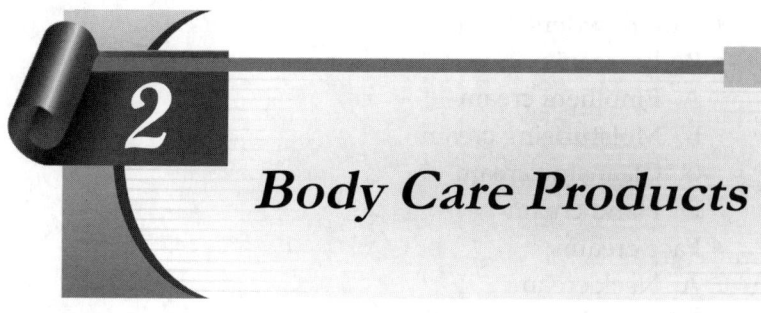

Body Care Products

Body care products generally consist of (a) body bath and (b) body massage oils. Skin forms the largest part of the body. Therefore, it is no surprise that it commands a considerable attention of skin care formulations.

In India, body massage is an age-old practice. Body massage oils and bath oils are popular products. Massage oils leave the skin surface oily. To cleanse the residual oil on the skin, bath is followed after massage. As a result bath powders were developed.

These bath powders especially herbal bath powders were developed with the dual purpose of keeping the body clean, fresh and pleasantly fragrant throughout the day. In addition, oil bath is a common practice once a week in this part of the world, to "overhaul" the body.

Body creams help in keeping the skin emollient, smooth and protect it from dry harsh weather. Face creams are to take care of wrinkles (wrinkle care) and complexion. There are of two types creams — o/w (oil in water) and w/o (water in oil).

Body care powders are mostly for body and face. Body care powders or talcum powders are generally used after bath to adsorb and absorb the residual moisture on the body.

Face powders are to cover the shine on the face and provide freshness.

Types of body care products:
- Body oils
- Face oils

- Bath powders
- Body creams
  A. Emollient cream
  B. Moisturising cream
  C. Cleansing cream
  D. Hand cream
- Face creams
  A. Neck cream
  B. Vanishing (cleansing cream)
  C. Anti-acne cream
- Body powders
  A. Talcum powder
  B. Prickly heat powder
  C. Aftershave powder
- Face powders

Table 2.1: Plants used in body care products

S. No.	Herbs	Parts used	Property
1.	Acacia concinna (Fig. 2.1)	Pods	Skin cleanser
2.	Aloe barbadensis (Fig. 2.2)	Leaves	Moisturiser
3.	Artabotrys odoratissimus (Fig. 2.3)	Flowers	Fragrance
4.	Artemesia vulgaris (Fig. 2.4)	Leaves	Skin protective
5.	Azadirachta indica (Fig. 2.5)	Leaves	Skin protective
6.	Berberis aristata (Fig. 2.6)	Roots	Skin protective
7.	Calendula officinalis (Fig. 2.7)	Flowers	Toning, complexion maintaining
8.	Carica papaya (Fig. 2.8)	Milk	Skin toning
9.	Chamecyparia obtusa (Fig. 2.9)	Flower extract	Fragrance, refreshing

(Contd.)

(Contd.)

10.	*Citrus limon* (Fig. 2.10)	Rinds	Fragrance, freshening
11.	*Curcuma longa* (Fig. 2.11)	Rhizomes	Skin protective
12.	*Curcuma aromatica* (Fig. 2.12)	Rhizomes	Fragrance, freshening
13.	*Curcuma zedoaria* (Fig. 2.13)	Rhizomes	Fragrance, freshening
14.	*Cyperus rotandus* (Fig. 2.14)	Roots	Fragrance, refreshing
15.	*Epiphyllum oxypetalum* (Fig. 2.15)	Flowers	Fragrance
16.	*Hemidesmus indicus* (Fig. 2.16)	Roots	Blending the perfume
17.	*Mimusops elengi* (Fig. 2.17)	Flowers	Fragrance, freshening
18.	*Ocimum basilicum* (Fig. 2.18)	Leaves	Skin protective
19.	*Pandanus odoratissimus* (Fig. 2.19)	Leaves	Fragrance, freshening
20.	*Pelargonium peltatum* (Fig. 2.20)	Leaves	Perfume enhancer
21.	*Plumbago indica* (Fig. 2.21)	Roots	Skin protective
22.	*Prunus amygdalus* (Fig. 2.22)	Seed oil	Cleansing, complexion improving
23.	*Psoralea cordifolia* (Fig. 2.23)	Seeds	Skin protective, melanin balancer
24.	*Pterocarpus santalinus* (Fig. 2.24)	Trunk	Protective, scar care
25.	*Rosa louise odier* (Fig. 2.25)	Flowers	Fragrance, astringent
26.	*Rubia cordifolia* (Fig. 2.26)	Stem	Protective, complexion maintaining
27.	*Santalum album* (Fig. 2.27)	Bark	Complexion improving, freshening
28.	*Sapindus mukorossi* (Fig. 2.28)	Roots	Skin cleanser
29.	*Vetiveria zizanioides* (Fig. 2.29)	Roots	Fragrance, cooling

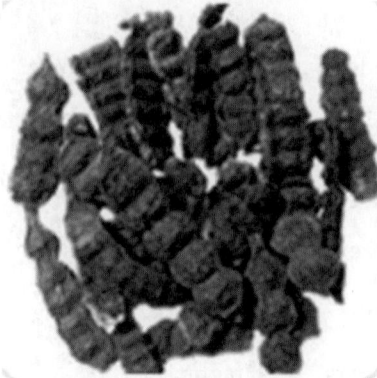

Fig. 2.1: *Acacia concinna*

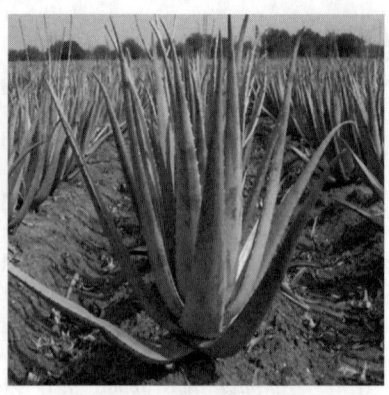

Fig. 2.2: *Aloe barbadensis*

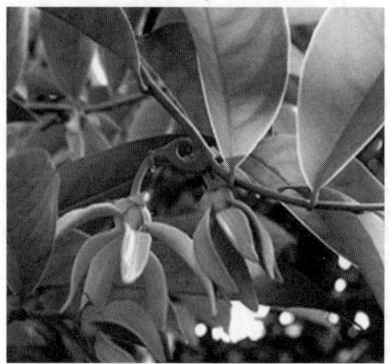

Fig. 2.3: *Artabotrys odoratissimus*

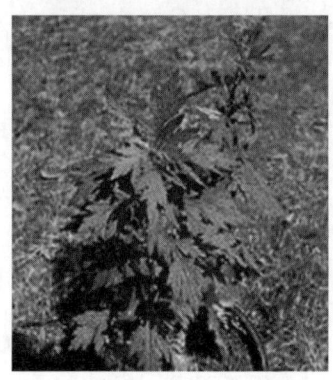

Fig. 2.4: *Artemesia vulgaris*

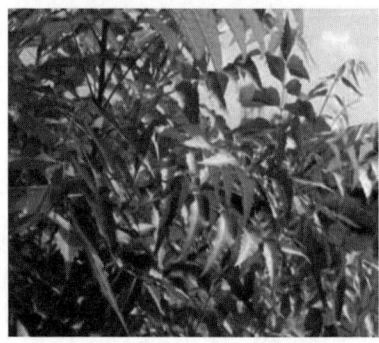

Fig. 2.5: *Azadirachta indica*

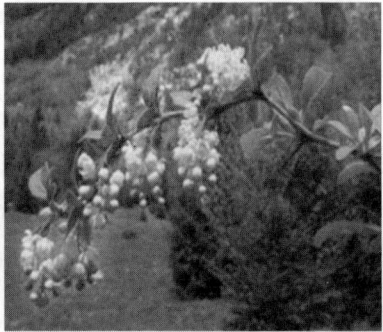

Fig. 2.6: *Berberis aristata*

Fig. 2.7: *Calendula officinalis*

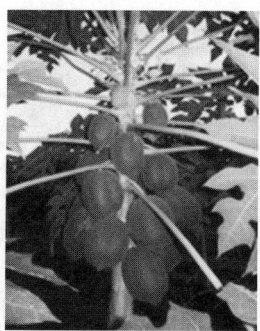

Fig. 2.8: *Carica papaya*

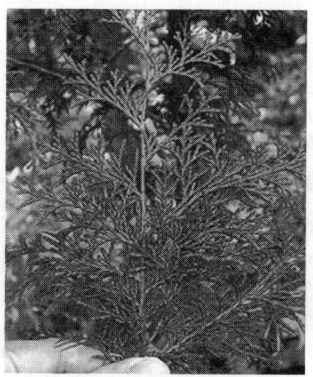

Fig. 2.9: *Chamecyparia obtusa*

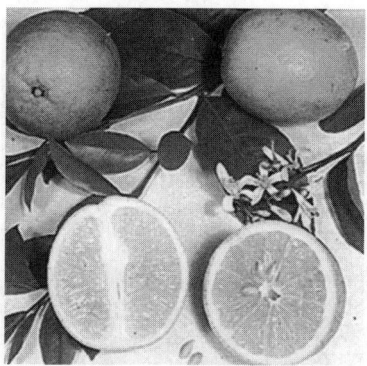

Fig. 2.10: *Citrus limon*

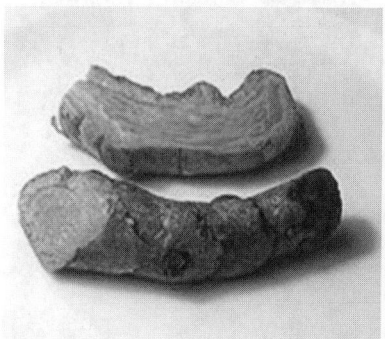

Fig. 2.11: *Curcuma longa*

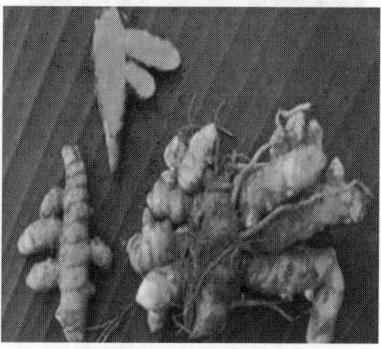

Fig. 2.12: *Curcuma aromatica*

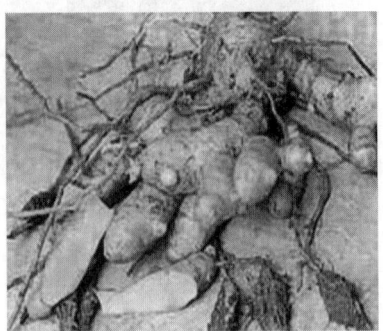

Fig. 2.13: *Curcuma zedoaria*

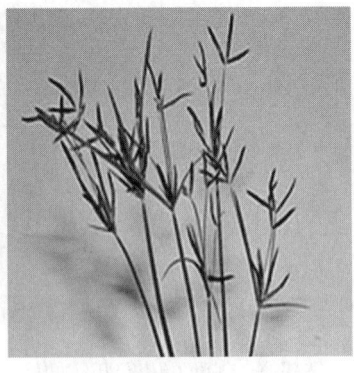

Fig. 2.14: *Cyperus rotandus*

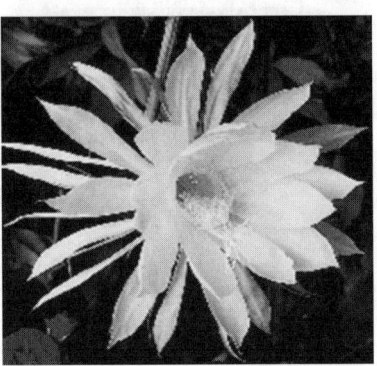

Fig. 2.15: *Epiphyllum oxypetalum*

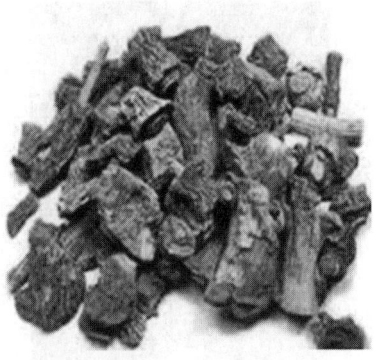

Fig. 2.16: *Hemidesmus indicus*

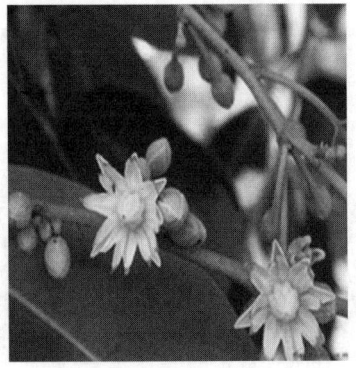

Fig. 2.17: *Mimusops elengi*

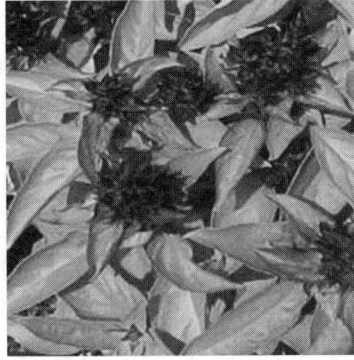

Fig. 2.18: *Ocimum basilicum*

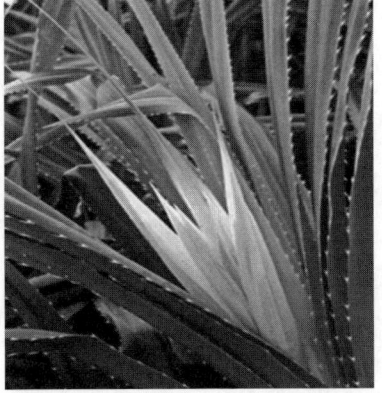

Fig. 2.19: *Pandanus odoratissimus*

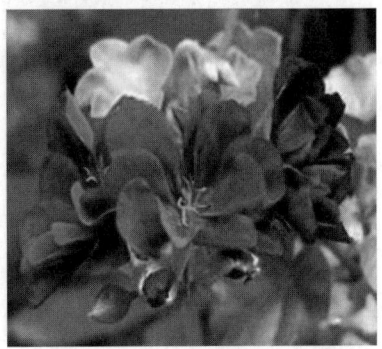

Fig. 2.20: *Pelargonium peltatum*

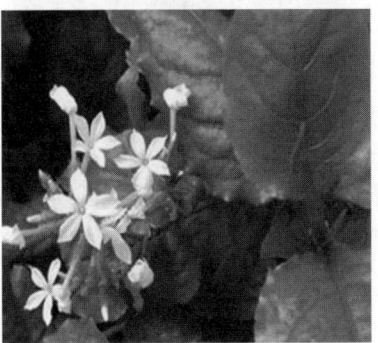

Fig. 2.21: *Plumbago indica*

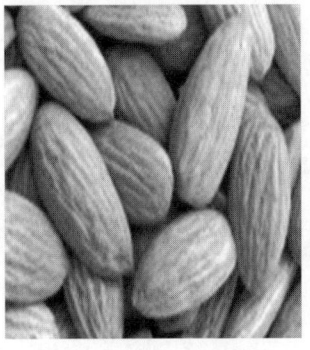

Fig. 2.22: *Prunus amygdalus*

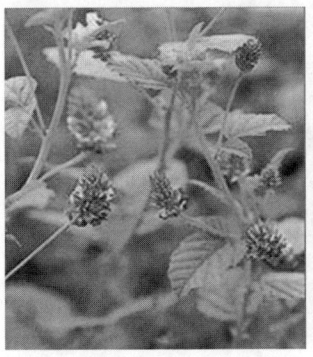

Fig. 2.23: *Psoralea cordifolia*

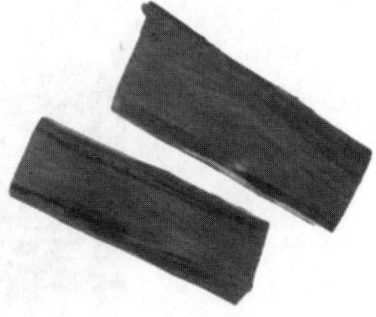

Fig. 2.24: *Pterocarpus santalinus*

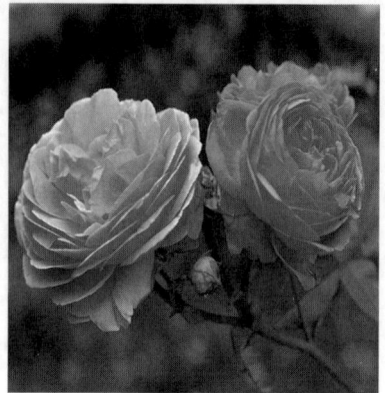

Fig. 2.25: *Rosa louise odier*

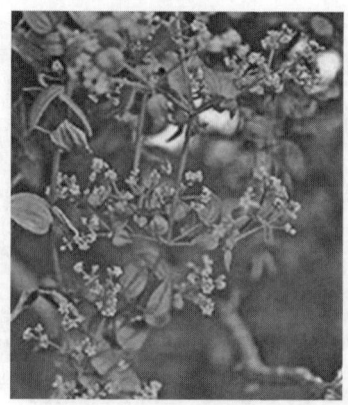

Fig. 2.26: *Rubia cordifolia*

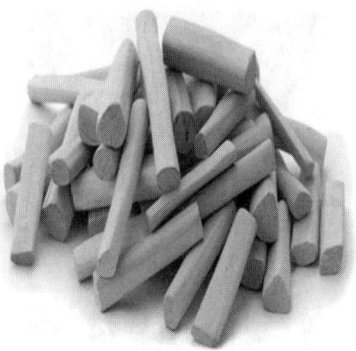

Fig. 2.27: *Santalum album*

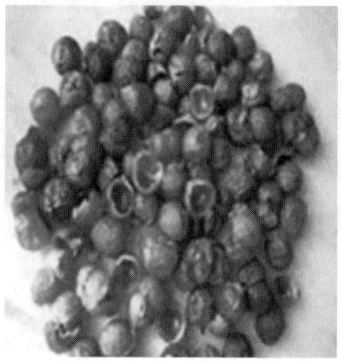

Fig. 2.28: *Sapindus mukorossi*

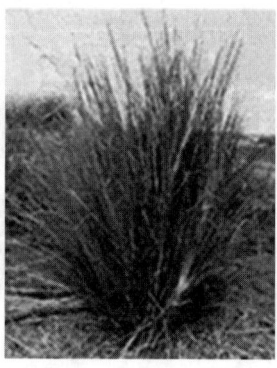

Fig. 2.29: *Vetiveria zizanioides*

BODY MASSAGE OILS

Oil massage to the body, followed by bath with bath powders once in a week is an age-old practice in India. This is to help cleanse the body, invigorate and refresh it. Body massage oils impart muscle relaxation, nourishing and toning up of muscles and also improve blood circulation. A blend of 2–3 vegetable oils is generally the practice. Mustard oil, sunflower oil, coconut oil and til oil are commonly used.

Bath Oil Forte/Massage Oil Forte

To impart more benefits to ordinary bath oil, a few essential oils, e.g. nutmeg, eucalyptus and thymol are added sometimes in order to make it a more invigorating one.

Formulations

Table 2.2

S. No.	Base Ingredient	%	S. No.	Herbal extracts mix Ingredient	Parts
1.	Sesame oil	40	1.	Azadirachta indica	5
2.	Mustard oil	10	2.	Curcuma aromatica	3
3.	Coconut oil	20	3.	Psoralea cordifolia	2
4.	Almond oil	10	4.	Berberis aristata	2
5.	Olive oil	20	5.	Cyprus rotandus	5
			6.	Thespesia purpurea	3

Table 2.3

S. No.	Base Ingredient	%	S. No.	Herbal extracts mix Ingredient	Parts
1.	Til oil	80	1.	Azadirachta indica	5
2.	Mustard oil	10	2.	Curcuma aromatica	3
3.	Coconut oil	10	3.	Psoralea cordifolia	2
			4.	Santalum album	1
			5.	Cyprus rotandus	5
			6.	Vetiveria zizanioides	3
			7.	Mimusops elengi	4
			8.	Cassia fistula	3

Table 2.4

Base			Herbal extracts mix		
S. No.	Ingredient	%	S. No.	Ingredient	Parts
1.	Til oil	60	1.	Azadirachta indica	5
2.	Mustard oil	15	2.	Curcuma aromatica	3
3.	Coconut oil	5	3.	Psoralea cordifolia	2
4.	Olive oil	5	4.	Berberis aristata	2
5.	Eucalyptus oil	5	5.	Cyprus rotandus	5
6.	Thymol	5	6.	Thespesia purpurea	3
7.	Nutmeg oil	5	7.	Matricaria recutita	2

About 5–10 ml of the blended oil is normally used depending on where it is to be applied. It helps in increasing the circulation of blood and growth of the muscles as stimulants and also to keep the skin tender, lustrous and toned.

Manufacturing

All the oils and herbal extract mix are raised to 70°C and heated under low fire for 5 minutes and then transferred to SS storage tanks. These massage oils are sometimes mixed with essential oils like nutmeg, lavender, thymol and eucalyptus.

FACE OILS

Achieving facial beauty is the prime goal for the formulators of facial cosmetics. It is the psychology of human beings that the face should ever look tender, youthful and wrinkle free. Our ancestors used many facial beauty preparations including facial massage oils. Raw turmeric paste in the colloidal form was and is popular among ladies. Turmeric paste will help as a depilatory, to impart smoothness to the skin, as a protective, antiseptic and help in improving the complexion of the skin. Apart from *Berberis aristata, Psoralia cordifolia* seeds, *Hemidesmus indicus* and *Azadirachta indica* are the herbs that help in imparting the desired effects discussed above to the facial skin. The facial massage oils are prepared from the extracts of these herbs in different combinations.

Oils that are helpful for the desired qualities as mentioned are:

1. Almond oil
2. Til oil
3. Cotton seed oil
4. Coconut oil
5. Sunflower oil

Table 2.5

Base			Herbal extracts mix		
S. No.	Ingredient	%	S. No.	Ingredient	Parts
1.	Til oil	40	1.	Curcuma longa	5
2.	Cotton seed oil	25	2.	Curcuma aromatica	3
3.	Sunflower oil	35	3.	Calendula officinalis	2
4.	Perfume	QS	4.	Azadirachta indica (flowers)	4

Table 2.6

Base			Herbal extracts mix		
S. No.	Ingredient	%	S. No.	Ingredients	Parts
1.	Almond oil	70	1.	Berberis aristata	5
2.	Til oil	20	2.	Hemidesmus indicus	5
3.	Wheat germ oil	5	3.	Asparagus racemosus	5
4.	Ruta graveolens	5	4.	Water	20
5.	Perfume	QS			

Manufacturing

All the oils are mixed and boiled with the extracts till the end product becomes clear. It is then kept in SS storage tank for 24 hours, filtered and bottled.

Quality Control

All the raw materials specially the vegetable oils are to be checked and analysed for each batch such that consistency in the finished product is uniform. The manufactured product should be:

1. Crystal clear

2. Free from moisture

The essential oils help in keeping the skin fragrant, fresh and provide a protective coat on the skin.

Specific gravity, refractive index, viscosity (80 cps), to name a few, tests should be conducted to maintain the desired consistency and batch to batch uniformity.

Preservation

As the oils are all vulnerable to rancidity, it is preferable to add about 2% antioxidants as preservatives for longer shelf life and maintaining the quality of the product.

Packing and Storage

Stored in bottles away from light and heat.

Evaluation

The oil should be lubricating and should not leave a heavy residual film after massage. The oil should more or less be completely absorbed by the skin after a little massage leaving a very thin film on the skin.

BODY BATH POWDERS

Bath powders are used to cleanse the body. As discussed earlier, oil bath is a tradition in India. After applying massage oil to the body (head and body) once in every week for ten minutes, the bath powder is made into a semisolid paste with water and applied to the body and then removed along with the body oil by washing.

Formulations

Table 2.7

Base			Herbal extracts mix		
S. No.	Ingredient	%	S. No.	Ingredient	Parts
1.	Bengal gram flour	60	1.	Michalea champa petals	5
2.	Green gram flour	20	2.	Santalum album powder	5
3.	Rice flour	10	3.	Curcuma zedoaria	5
4.	Acacia concinna rita	5	4.	Vetiveria zizanioides	5
5.	Celite	5	5.	Psoralea cordifolia	10
			6.	Artemesia vulgaris	10
			7.	Azadirachta indica leaf	10
			8.	Mimusops elengi flowers	3
			9.	Acacia concinna	2

Table 2.8

Base			Herbal extracts mix		
S. No.	Ingredient	%	S. No.	Ingredient	Parts
1.	Bengal gram flour	40	1.	Azadirachta indica leaf	5
2.	Green gram flour	40	2.	Santalum album powder	3
3.	Celite	15	3.	Acacia concinna	4
4.	Multani mitti	5	4.	Curcuma zedoaria	1
			5.	Psoralea cordifolia	4

Table 2.9

Base			Herbal extracts mix		
S. No.	Ingredient	%	S. No.	Ingredient	Parts
1.	Bengal gram flour	60	1.	Azadirachta indica leaf	8
2.	Green gram flour	25	2.	Santalum album powder	3
3.	Rice flour	5	3.	Vetiveria zizanioides	3
4.	Multani mitti	5	4.	Cyprus rotandus	4
5.	Kiesulguhr	5	5.	Mimusops elengi	5
			6.	Michalea champa	5
			7.	Curcuma aromatica	1
			8.	Curcuma zedoaria	3

Table 2.10

Base			Herbal extracts mix		
S. No.	Ingredient	%	S. No.	Ingredient	Parts
1.	Bengal gram flour	50	1.	Ficus bengalensis	5
2.	Green gram flour	40	2.	Curcuma zedoaria	10
3.	Multani mitti	10	3.	Azadirachta indica	5
4.	Preservatives	QS		leaf	

Manufacturing

The base is mixed with the herbal powder mix and blended in a double cone blender for half an hour and sifted through 80 mesh sieve to get a smooth powder free from gritty or fibrous particles and packed.

Quality Control

The powder should pass through 80 mesh sieve freely.

Packing and Storage

The powder is filled in polyethylene bags, sealed and packed in an outer carton or a container and stored away from light and heat.

Evaluation

After bathing with this powder, the skin of the body should be free from grease and any residual dirt and fresh and fragrant.

BODY CREAMS

Mostly massage creams are emollients also. These body massage creams are made out of herbal massage oil, water and emulsifiers. They are skin food and toners. In addition, the herbs help in adding protective properties to the skin. Herbal massage creams are also muscle relaxants.

Body creams help in keeping the skin emollient and smooth and protect from dry harsh weather. There are two types of creams—o/w (oil in water) and w/o (water in oil). For a body massage, the o/w cream is made with vegetable oils, herbal massage oils and herbal extracts. The o/w type is helpful for massage as it imparts lubrication and opens the pores of the skin after massage.

The second type w/o is used for nourishing the skin and as a foundation cream for make up. The herbal extracts in the formula are broadly included for the purpose of nourishing.

Emollient Cream

Emollient creams provide water to stratum corneum on application and keep the skin smooth and free from dryness.

Formulations

Table 2.11

Non-aqueous phase (oily)			Aqueous phase		
S. No.	Ingredient	%	S. No.	Ingredient	Parts
1.	Glyceryl mono stearate (GMS)	12	1.	Propylene glycol	7
			2.	Duponol C	0.5
2.	Petrolatum, white USP	4	3.	Water	60
3.	Almond oil	8	4.	D and C orange	0.05
4.	Herbal extracts	5		No. 4, 1%	
5.	Stearic acid	3	5.	Methyl paraben	0.15
6.	Cocoa butter	1			

Herbal extracts mix		
S. No.	Ingredient	Parts
1.	Pelargonium peltatum	2
2.	Rosa louise odier	1
3.	Jasminum grandiflorum	3

Manufacturing

Mix the herbal extracts in the aqueous phase and preservatives and mix A and B at 75°C. Stir well before feeding into colloid mill. Pass through the colloid mill and transfer it into a SS tank to congeal at 45°C. After the cream is set, fill it and pack.

Quality Control

Penetrability and spreadability: 1 g/10 sq.cm. and viscosity 6000 cps.

Storage

Store the material in a cool and dry place.

Evaluation

Mild absorption in the skin with minimum quantity of application. This cream should impart softness, smoothness to the skin and protect it from roughness.

Moisturising Cream

Moisturising creams are generally used to protect the skin from scaling by providing adequate hydration.

Table 2.12

Oil phase			Aqueous phase		
S. No.	Ingredient	%	S. No.	Ingredient	Parts
1.	Coconut oil	50	1.	Water	30
2.	Stearic acid	2	2.	Herbal extracts	4
3.	Cetyl alcohol	2	3.	Preservatives	QS
4.	Isopropyl myristate	3	4.	Perfume	QS
5.	Glyceryl stearate	2			
6.	PEG 100 stearate	3			
7.	Lanolin hydrous	2			
8.	Shea butter	2			

S. No.	Herbal extracts mix Ingredient	Parts
1.	*Aloe barbadensis*	0.2
2.	*Matricaria recutita*	3.0
3.	*Citrus limon*	0.1
4.	*Citrus aurantium* peel	0.1

Table 2.13

Oil phase S. No.	Ingredient	%	Aqueous phase S. No.	Ingredient	%
1.	Hydrogenated coconut oil	22	1.	Water	60
2.	Glyceryl stearate	2	2.	Sorbitol	5
3.	Cetyl alcohol	1	3.	Triethanolamine	3
4.	Cocoa butter	2	4.	Antioxidant	1
			5.	PEG cocoamine	4
			6.	Perfume	QS
			7.	Preservatives	QS

S. No.	Herbal extracts mix Ingredient	Parts
1.	*Artabotrys odoratissimus*	2
2.	*Chamecyparia obtusa*	2
3.	*Aloe barbadensis*	2

Manufacturing

Mix the herbal extracts in the aqueous phase, A and B ingredients are heated separately to 70°C and stirred till the mass congeals at 40°C.

Table 2.14

Non-aqueous phase (oily)			Aqueous phase		
S. No.	Ingredient	%	S. No.	Ingredient	%
1.	Triple pressed stearic acid	2	1.	Water	75
2.	Cetyl alcohol	2	2.	Herbal extracts mix	6
3.	Isopropyl myristate	2	3.	Perfume	QS
4.	Wool fat hydrous glyceryl stearate	10	4.	Preservatives	QS
5.	PEG 100 stearate	3			

Herbal extracts mix		
S. No.	Ingredient	Parts
1.	Artabotrys odoratissimus	2
2.	Chamecyparia obtusa	2
3.	Aloe barbadensis	2

Mix the herbal extracts in the aqueous phase, A and B are heated up to 70°C and stirred after mixing together for 15 minutes till it congeals. Fill into containers and pack.

Table 2.15

Non-aqueous phase (oily)			Aqueous phase		
S. No.	Ingredient	%	S. No.	Ingredient	%
1.	Stearic acid, (triple pressed)	2	1.	Water	74.5
2.	Cetyl alcohol	2	2.	Glycerin	4
3.	Isopropyl myristate	2	3.	Triethanolamine	1
4.	Lanolin oil	10	4.	Preservatives	QS
5.	Glyceryl stearate	1.5			
6.	PEG 100 stearate	1.5			
7.	Magnesium aluminium silicate	1.5			

Herbal extracts mix		
S. No.	Ingredient	Parts
1.	Aloe barbadensis	2
2.	Michalia alba	2

Manufacturing

Mix the herbal extracts in the aqueous phase, A and B are heated up to 70°C and stirred after mixing together for 15 minutes till it congeals. Fill into containers and pack.

Quality Control

Viscosity 8000 cps, spreadability 1 g/15 sq. m. of the skin area.

Evaluation

It should impart moisture to the skin and make the skin free from dryness.

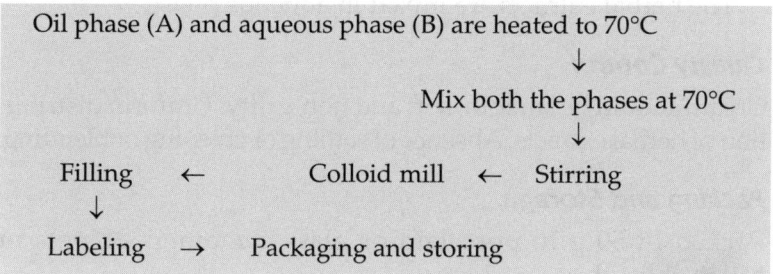

Fig. 2.30: Scheme/flow sheet

Cleansing Cream

This is a non-massage type mainly with stearic acid, soap wax and only as an application on the body before talcum powder.

Table 2.16

Non-aqueous phase (oily)			Aqueous phase		
S. No.	Ingredient	%	S. No.	Ingredient	%
1.	Carnuba wax	3	1.	Water	67
2.	Hydrolysed proteins from almonds	6	2.	Monoethanolamine	3
3.	Stearyl alcohol	3	3.	Propylene glycol	8
4.	Glyceryl stearate	3	4.	Sodium dehydro acetate	2
5.	Coconut oil	2			
6.	Triethanolamine stearate	3			

Herbal extracts mix		
S. No.	Ingredient	Parts
1.	Acacia concinna	2
2.	Phaseolus aureus	2
3	Artemesia pallense	2
4	Artemesia vulgaris	3

Manufacturing

A and B phases are heated up to 70°C and stirred after mixing both the phases at 70°C. Stirring is continued till the mass is congealed at room temperature.

The herbal extracts are mixed in aqueous phase.

Quality Control

Cream should be smooth, soft and non-gritty. Uniform distribution of herbal extracts. Absence of settling or creeping or blending.

Packing and Storage

Packed in 50 g in porcelain or glass containers or pots or collapsible tubes.

Evaluation

Cleanse the area wherever it is applied on the body skin.

Hand Cream

Hand creams are used to keep the hands free from dryness, "denaturing" of the skin and keep it smooth and soft.

Table 2.17

Non-aqueous phase (oily)			Aqueous phase		
S. No.	Ingredient	%	S. No.	Ingredient	%
1.	Cetyl alcohol	3	1.	Water	75
2.	Glyceryl monostearate	3	2.	Sodium hydroxide	5
3.	Isopropyl palmitate	7	3.	Aloe vera	2
4.	Lanolin	2			
5.	Til oil	2			
6.	PEG 1000 monostearate	1			

Herbal extracts mix		
S. No.	*Ingredient*	*Parts*
1.	*Artabotrys odoratissimus*	3
2.	*Artemisia nilgririka*	2

Manufacturing

Heat the aqueous and non-aqueous phases to 70°C. Mix the two phases and stir till the mixture congeals.

Quality Control

The cream should be smooth and spreadable easily when applied to hands and finally absorbed, leaving moisture on the hands and not an oily residue. Spreadability should be reproducible and uniform for all batches. There should not be any variation from batch to batch.

Preservation

A combination of methyl and propyl paraben.

Safety and Efficacy

The base chemicals that are selected in the formula are all free from side effects or any other harmful effects. Hence, the cream is safe.

Storage

Stored in a cool place away from light at room temperature.

Evaluation

Hands are to be free from dryness and brittleness, keeping the hands soft and smooth.

FACE CREAMS

The purpose of face creams is to take care of wrinkles (wrinkle care) and complexion. Facial massage creams are generally o/w type prepared out of vegetable oils, e.g. almond oil and apricot oil and they help in taking care of the facial skin, by providing an anti-wrinkle effect and glow to the facial skin.

Table 2.18

Non-aqueous phase (oily)			Aqueous phase		
S. No.	*Ingredient*	*%*	*S. No.*	*Ingredient*	*%*
1.	Almond oil	30	1.	Water	30
2.	Apricot oil	28	2.	Borax	3
3.	Stearic acid	2	3.	Triethanolamine	2
4.	Beeswax	3	4.	Carbopol	0.5
5.	Cocoa butter	1.5	5.	Perfume	QS
			6.	Preservatives	QS

Herbal extracts mix		
S. No.	*Ingredient*	*Parts*
1.	*Tagetes erecta*	2
2.	*Rosa louise odier*	3
3.	*Curcuma aromatica*	2
4.	*Berberis aristata*	3

Vanishing Cream (Cleansing Cream)

These are bases for foundation in make up and only for external application without massage, for spreading on the skin. Hence, no oil phase is necessary. The soap helps in cleansing the skin additionally and freshening.

Table 2.19

Non-aqueous phase (oily)			Aqueous phase		
S. No.	*Ingredient*	*%*	*S. No.*	*Ingredient*	*%*
1.	Cyclomethicone	3.6	1.	Water	91.2
2.	Stearic acid	1.4	2.	Glycerin	2.0
3.	Cetyl alcohol	1.0	3.	Triethanolamine	0.8

Herbal extracts mix		
S. No.	*Ingredient*	*Parts*
1.	*Psoralea cordifolia*	3
2.	*Santalum album* oil	0.1
3.	*Curcuma aromatica*	2
4.	*Glycyrrhiza glabra*	2

Manufacturing

Mix both phases (i) oily phase and (ii) aqueous phase at 70°C and stir with a mechanical stirrer and then pass through colloid mill before it is transferred to SS storage tanks and then stored for 48 hours before packaging.

Quality Control

The cream should be uniform in texture. It should spread easily when applied on the skin. Minimum quantity with maximum area coverage (spreading) should not clog the pores of the skin. Perfume should last throughout the shelf life. Viscosity 8000 cps, spreadability and penetrability.

Preservation and Storage

These creams can be preserved, when they are stored away from light at room temperature and with addition of preservatives up to about 24 months.

Evaluation

Cleansing of the skin, should not clog the pores of the skin and skin freshening.

Anti-acne Cream

Acne is invariably associated with adolescence. Several anti-acne creams are available in the market. However, anti-acne herbal creams are much sought after these days as they are relatively safer. Regular application of these creams restores normalcy to the facial skin without any ugly scars.

Table 2.20

Base				Herbal extracts mix		
S. No.	Ingredient	%		S. No.	Ingredient	Parts
1.	Bentonite	13		1.	Rubia cordifolia	3
2.	Soft paraffin	10		2.	Pterocarpus marsupium	3
3.	Cotton seed oil	6		3.	Azadirachta indica	2
4.	Glycerin	12				
5.	Water	55				
6.	Borax	4				
7.	Preservatives	QS				
8.	Perfume	QS				

Manufacturing

Bentonite is soaked in water for about 24 hours depending on the water number capacity of bentonite. Cotton seed oil is mixed with soft paraffin and heated. Herbal extract mix is dissolved in a portion of water and heated simultaneously. The oil phase is slowly introduced into the bentonite and mixed to form a base. Then water with extract heated to about 65°C is added and the mixture is homogenised, after adding the preservatives and perfume.

Quality Control

All the herbs must be pure and of high quality with reproducible analytical data to ensure quality of the end product. All the raw materials must be free from microbes.

Packing and Storage

Packed in either collapsible tubes or HDPE jars and stored in a cool and dry place.

Evaluation

Spreadability, penetration, absorption, proper adherence.

Herbal Surma—Eyelid Cream (Kajal)

Two plants are traditionally used to make kajal.
1. Eclipta alba, and
2. Punica granatum.

Herbs

1. Eclipta alba — leaf juice
2. Punica granatum — seed juice

Ingredients

1. Castor oil
2. Cotton wick
3. Butter

Manufacturing

A cotton wick is dipped in castor oil and burnt till soot is formed and collected on a reversed silver or copper plate covered over the wick. The wick is first soaked in *Eclipta alba*—leaf juice and *Punica granatum*—seed juice overnight and dried. This dried wick is dipped second time in castor oil and burnt to collect the soot formed in closed air with silver or copper plate. This soot is further collected and mixed with butter to get a paste.

Quality Control

Consistency, viscosity, fluidity, sufficient to keep the paste at the site of application.

Fine and smooth paste without any gritty particles.

Should not run off the site.

Herbal Lipstick

Herbs used are *Nyctanthes arbortristis* flower stalks extract, which gives an orange red—dye.

Herbs

1. *Nyctanthes arbortristis* flower stalks.

Ingredients

1. Castor oil
2. Beeswax

Manufacturing

The beeswax and castor oil are put together, warmed up to 60°C and the colour is added. When the temperature is 50°C stirred once again, set aside for 24 hours after pouring in the moulds. The natural dye obtained from Nyctanthes flower stalks is safe and harmless.

Neck Cream

Neck creams are specially made for masking the wrinkles of neck muscles.

Table 2.21

Non-aqueous phase (oily)		
S. No.	Ingredient	%
1.	Sunflower oil with vitamins A and E	23
2.	Stearyl alcohol	2
3.	Lanolin	2
4.	Zinc stearate	1
5.	Dioctyl succinate	2
6.	Myrstyl myristate	3
7.	Lanolin alcohol	2
8.	Magnesium aluminium silicate	2
9.	Retinyl palmitate	5

Aqueous phase		
S. No.	Ingredient	%
1.	Water	48
2.	Glycol stearate	2
3.	Myrstyl myristate	3
4.	Wool alcohol	5

Herbal extracts mix		
S. No.	Ingredient	Parts
1.	Aloe barbadensis	2
2.	Moringa olefera	3

Manufacturing

Both A and B phases are heated up to 70°C and stirred in a manufacturing vessel for 15 minutes and then transferred to a colloid mill. When it starts congealing, it is emptied into a S.S. storage tank.

Quality Control

Cream should be smooth, soft and non-gritty.

Packing and Storage

Packed into unit dosage form like 50 g in porcelain or glass containers or pots or collapsible tubes.

Evaluation

Neck muscles should get toned up without sagging, should mask wrinkles if any.

BODY POWDERS

These are generally the talcum powders used after bath to adsorb and absorb the residual moisture on the body in order to keep the body dry, fresh and fragrant. The second variety is prickly heat dusting powders widely used in tropical countries, to take care of perspiration, which leads to small eruptions on the skin called prickly heat.

Formulations

Table 2.22

Base			Herbal extracts mix		
S. No.	Ingredient	%	S. No.	Ingredient	Parts
1.	Talc	80	1.	Azadirachta indica	8
2.	Zinc stearate	2	2.	Santalum album	3
3.	Precipitated chalk	8	3.	Vetiveria zizanioides	2
4.	Herbal powders mix	10	4.	Chamecyparia obutusa	3
			5.	Cyprus rotandus	4

Table 2.23

Base			Herbal extracts mix		
S. No.	Ingredient	%	S. No.	Ingredient	Parts
1.	Talc	70	1.	Azadirachta indica	
2.	Zinc stearate	6	2.	Santalum album	3
3.	Rice starch	3	3.	Artemesia vulgaris	3
4.	Precipitated chalk	8	4.	Cyprus rotandus	4
5.	Magnesium carbonate	5	5.	Chamecyparia obutusa	3
6.	Herbal powder mix	8	6.	Psoralia cordifolia	3
7.	Perfume—sandal	QS	7.	Curcuma aromatica	2
			8.	Curcuma zedoaria	3

Table 2.24

Base			Herbal extracts mix		
S. No.	Ingredient	%	S. No.	Ingredient	Parts
1.	Talc	50	1.	Artemesia vulgaris	3
2.	Zinc oxide	12	2.	Santalum album	2
3.	Magnesium carbonate	10	3.	Curcuma aromatica	2
4.	Zinc stearate	5	4.	Pandanus odoratissimus	2
5.	Rice starch	10			
6.	Precipitated chalk	5			
7.	Herbal powders mix	8			

Dusting Powders

Table 2.25

Base			Herbal extracts mix		
S. No.	Ingredient	%	S. No.	Ingredient	Parts
1.	Kaolin or fine Kieselguhr	25	1.	Azadirachta indica	3
2.	Talc	50	2.	Tagetus erecta	2
3.	Precipated chalk	25	3.	Berberis aristata	2
4.	Perfume—lavender	QS			

Manufacturing

The choice perfume is mixed with magnesium carbonate thoroughly then the base, before herbal powder mix is blended with the base mixture.

Quality Control

Quality is checked for adherence and covering. Perfume stability and degree of fragrance is also noted. The fragrance should be maintained same by the powder throughout the shelf life from the date of manufacturing

Packing and Storage

Stored in tightly closed tin containers in a cool dry place.

Evaluation

Free flow

Prickly Heat Powders

Prickly heat occurs on the skin due to profuse perspiration, generally in summer resulting in an eruption which gives discomfort
to the individual with pruritus and scratching. Prickly heat
powders offer relief from itching.

Table 2.26

S. No.	Base Ingredient	%	S. No.	Herbal extracts mix Ingredient	Parts
1.	Talc	50	1.	Azadirachta indica	4
2.	Zinc oxide	30	2.	Ocimum basilicum	2
3.	Rice starch	5	3.	Santalum album	3
4.	Magnesium carbonate	5	4.	Vetiveria zizanioides	5
5.	Herbal mix	10	5.	Camphor	3
6.	Colour	QS			

Table 2.27

S. No.	Base Ingredient	%	S. No.	Herbal extracts mix Ingredient	Parts
1.	Talc	70	1.	Azadirachta indica leaf	8
2.	Zinc stearate	6	2.	Santalum album	3
3.	Rice starch	3	3.	Vetiveria zizanioides	2
4.	Precipitate chalk	8	4.	Camphor	3
5.	Magnesium carbonate	5			
6.	Herbal powder mix	8			
7.	Perfume (sandal)	QS			

Table 2.28

S. No.	Base Ingredient	%	S. No.	Herbal extracts mix Ingredient	Parts
1.	Talc	40	1.	Santalum album	4
2.	Zinc oxide	8	2.	Azadirachta indica leaf	3
3.	Rice starch	7	3.	Camphor	3
4.	Precipitated chalk	10	4.	Ocimum basilicum	2
5.	Magnesium carbonate	15			
6.	Zinc stearate	15			
7.	Herbal powder mix	5			
8.	Perfume	QS			

Manufacturing

All the ingredients of base powders are sieved through 120 mesh and mixed/blended in a double cone blender. Lastly the herbal powder mix is added and blended thoroughly.

Quality Control

Degree of fineness and colour blending should be uniform. Colours should not bleed out when applied on the face.

Evaluation

Colour blending should be uniform

Packing and Storage

Stored in tightly closed tin containers in a cool dry place.

Aftershave Powder

Antiseptic/dusting powders are protective in nature in addition to good spreadability. Aftershave powders are mostly antiseptic and cooling to counter the irritation on a freshly shaven facial skin and provide comfort.

Table 2.29

Base			Herbal extracts mix		
S. No.	Ingredient	%	S. No.	Ingredient	Parts
1.	Talc	73	1.	Artemesia vulgaris	5
2.	Zinc stearate	2	2.	Ocimum basilicum	5
3.	Precipitated chalk	20	3.	Berberis aristata	3
4.	Zinc carbonate	1	4.	Mimusops elengi	2
5.	Magnesium carbonate	3	5.	Cressacreta	2
6.	Menthol	1			
7.	Perfume (lavender)	QS			

Manufacturing

All the above ingredients are mixed and blended in a double cone blender and passed through 100 mesh.

Quality Control

Uniformity in mixing and perfume should last throughout the shelf life.

Packing and Storage

Stored in tightly closed tin containers in a cool dry place.

Evaluation

The powder should adhere to the surface of the facial skin and spread uniformly.

FACE POWDERS

Face powder is a valuable cosmetic product for a common man. A large segment of people utilize it whereas body powders are used by a selective segment. Presently herbal face powder finds itself in a similar situation. But it would not be long before it attracts a larger segment of users.

The purpose of a face powder is to absorb the shine on the face and to give it a fresh appearance. A majority of powders contain talcum powder, magnesium carbonate and zinc oxide.

Face powders are formulated mainly keeping in mind the women folk. A woman's choice in selecting a face powder firstly hovers around its perfume, followed by:

1. Colour
2. Spreadability or coverage
3. Removal or management of shine on the face.

Face powder is the final item in the make up of a woman, after the foundation cream which helps in covering the minor defects on the face.

The facial skin is broadly categorized as (i) oily and (ii) dry. Further the shine on it is classified as heavy, medium and light. It is very important for formulators of face powders to take into account the above mentioned aspects.

The talcum powder used as a base, has the tendency of blackening the face on prolonged usage or in other words tends to make the skin look dark and also tends to leave the skin rough.

Herbal face powders are developed, designed and formulated in such a way that all these undesirable qualities of cosmetic face powders are countered and help to keep the facial skin normal, tender and fresh. The rationale in selection of herbs should be accurate.

Desirable Qualities of a Herbal Face Powder

1. Covering power/masking the shine on the face.
2. Easy application, pleasant, soothing, acceptable perfume.
3. Minimum quantity to cover maximum area.
4. Good slip and adhesion.
5. Agreeable shade.
6. Perfume should have lingering qualities, throughout the shelf life as well as during usage by the customer.
7. Minimum frequency of application on the face.

Table 2.30: Colour—perfume compatibility of face powders

S. No.	Herbal perfume	Shade/colour
1.	Santalum album perfume	Pale brownish/body colour
2.	Rosa louise odier	Pale pink colour
3.	Pandanus odoratissimus	Creamish body colour
4.	Curcuma longa	Pale yellowish, pale yellow
5.	Jasminum grandiflorum, chameli or mogra	White
6.	Lavandula angustifolia	Liliac or pale violet, light ochre
7.	Nichanthes arbotristis	Pale brick red shade, light peach
8.	Mimusops elengi	Creamish white or cream

The compatibility of colour and perfume is very important for the formulation of a herbal face powder. The concept of herbal face powder is relatively new. The herbs that are mostly beneficial to the face skin are judiciously selected and included in the formulation, e.g. *Rosa louise odier, Calendula officinalis, Pandanus odoratissimus, Mimusops elengi, Michelia champaca, Chamecyparia obtusa, Curcuma aromatica.*

An Ideal Face Powder

1. It should conceal the shine and minor skin imperfections. This can be done by covering power of the face powder. If the ideal covering power is not obtained by a single ingredient, a blend of two ingredients can be thought off. Talc and stearates can do the job.

2. Good adhesiveness is a must as the powder should remain on the skin for a considerable length of time.

3. Perfume and colour should be universally acceptable and lasting.

Magnesium carbonate is an ideal carrier of both perfume and colour. The perfume should be adsorbed and retained in the powder throughout its shelf life.

The covering agent included in the formulation of face powders is to be proportional to the base, which is an inert material and pass through 300 mesh and it should be capable of exhibiting at least one or two properties enlisted above.

The types of skin are classified into four categories—dry, normal, moderately oily and very oily. Dry skin secretes very less oil and moisture. Therefore, it requires a powder with light covering power.

Normal and moderately oily skin, being more shiny, due to secretion of sebum requires a powder with more covering power.

Very oily skin requires a powder of heavy covering power due to high shine.

There are many people, especially women with generally dry skin and yet they suffer from oily foreheads, oily noses or oily chins. In such cases, different powders with different covering powers are simultaneously used.

Similarly, the choice of shade of the powder is a very personal choice. Further, the colours of the face powders can be different for day and night.

Formulations

Table 2.31

S. No.	Herbal extracts mix Ingredient	Parts
1.	*Rosa louise odier* petal powder	2
2.	*Pelargonium peltatum*	2
3.	*Jasminum grandiflorum*	2

Face powders in general constitute a majority of the materials given in the table above. The most commonly selected materials are precipitated chalk, magnesium carbonate, starch and purified kaolin. Starch is an important constituent, possessing many desired properties in the formulation of a face powder. But it is not favoured in USA due to its clinging properties, and its tendency to absorb moisture. But it exhibits a peachy effect which is desirable in some types of powders. Most of the French face powders do, however, contain rice, starch blended with precipitated chalk. Apparently a judicious combination of rice, starch and processed chalk is helpful in obtaining the desired properties in the end product.

Although a majority of face powders contain the above mentioned materials (Table 2.32), in order to contribute to the qualities of an ideal herbal face powder, the base or the vehicle of face powder should be compatible with the herbal ingredient, which is going to be blended into it.

The floral dust of:

1. Kewda (*Pandanus odoratissimus*) or
2. The shade dried pandan leaves powder or

Table 2.32: Face powder

S. No.	Material	Rationale of usage
1.	Talc	Slip
2.	Starch	Adhesiveness
3.	Metallic soaps	Slip, lubrication
4.	Calcium, zinc and magnesium stearate	Shining
5.	Zinc oxide, zinc sulfide	Shining
6.	Colloidal clay	Bodying agent
7.	Celite or purified kaolin	Covering power
8.	Precipitated chalk	Covering power
9.	Purified kaolin	Covering power
10.	Lithophone kaolin colloidal	Covering power
11.	Magnesium carbonate	Perfume retaining
12.	Titanium dioxide	Whitening
13.	Calcium sulphate	Whitening
14.	Magnesium oxide	Spreadability

3. Scented turmeric (*Curcuma aromatica*)

4. Sandalwood powder (*Santalum album*)

These are some of the well known herbal powders that feature in many herbal face powder formulations.

Raw Materials for the Base/Vehicle:

Zinc oxide: Finest, white or creamy white grade

Talc: Finest grade 99% should pass through 200 mesh

Zinc stearate: Creamy white or white, made out of triple pressed stearic acid and odorless.

Precipitated chalk: Light and whitest grade

Magnesium carbonate: Lightest and creamy white

Formulations

Table 2.33

S. No.	Herbal face powder	%
	Base	
1.	Zinc oxide	20
2.	Talc	50
3.	Zinc stearate	6
4.	Rice starch	6
5.	Precipitated chalk	8
6.	Herbal powder	10
7.	Perfume	QS

As discussed, rice starch is one of the desired natural ingredient but due to some undesired properties some countries like USA tend to avoid it but in Europe it is very much a part of face powder formulations. In India, being a tropical country, this is a desired material, due to its capacity to absorb perspiration leaving a peachy effect. The inclusion of titanium dioxide is ever increasing in the formulations as it has more covering power, it is neutral, its lustrous and finely compatible with colour shades.

All ingredients can be retained in the same ratio for different shades of colour except titanium dioxide. The covering power of titanium dioxide is five times more than that of zinc oxide.

But the secretions of face, may not allow the ingredient to be stable on the face. However, a blend of zinc oxide and titanium dioxide neutralize the undesired effects.

Table 2.34

Light powders			Herbal extracts mix		
S. No.	Ingredient	%	S. No.	Ingredient	Parts
1.	Zinc oxide	23	1.	Curcuma aromatica	2
2.	Starch	8	2.	Pandanus odoratissimus	3
3.	Talc	62			
4.	Zinc stearate	4			
5.	Magnesium carbonate	3			
6.	Perfume	QS			

Table 2.35

Medium heavy powder base		
S. No.	Ingredient	%
1.	Zinc oxide	32
2.	Zinc stearate	5
3.	Magnesium carbonate	3
4.	Talc	50
5.	Rice starch	10
6.	Perfume (rose)	QS
7.	Colour (ochre)	QS

Table 2.36

Light powder base		
S. No.	Ingredient	%
1.	Titanium dioxide	6
2.	Talc	80
3.	Zinc stearate	5
4.	Magnesium carbonate	5
5.	Purified Kieselguhr	4
6.	Colour (yellow)	QS
7.	Perfume	QS

Table 2.37

S. No.	Heavy powder base Ingredient	%
1.	Zinc oxide	22
2.	Titanium dioxide	3
3.	Talc	68
4.	Zinc stearate	4
5.	Magnesium carbonate	3
6.	Perfume (rose)	QS
	Colour (pink)	QS

Table 2.38

S. No.	Natural powder base Ingredient	%
1.	Precipitated chalk	60
2.	Talc	40
3.	Golden (ochre–turmeric)	QS
4.	Perfume	QS

Table 2.39

S. No.	Naturelle Ingredient	%
1.	Precipitated chalk	70
2.	Colour—Goldern ochre	24

Table 2.40(i)

S. No.	Additional base formulae Ingredient	%
1.	Zinc carbonate	22
2.	Precipitated chalk	73
3.	Rice starch	5
4.	Colour (cream)	QS
5.	Perfume (kewda)	QS

Table 2.40(ii)

S. No.	Ingredient	%
1.	Talc	40
2.	Colloidal clay	26
3.	Zinc oxide	8
4.	Zinc stearate	1
5.	Precipitated chalk	15
6.	Magnesium carbonate	10
7.	Perfume and colour	QS

Table 2.40(iii)

S. No.	Ingredient	%	%
1.	Talc	40	50
2.	Colloidal clay	20	20
3.	Zinc oxide	20	10
4.	Zinc stearate	4	10
5.	Precipitated chalk	8	5
6.	Magnesium carbonate	8	5
7.	Perfume and colour	QS	QS

Table 2.40(iv)

S. No.	Ingredient	%
1.	Talc	70
2.	Zinc oxide	20
3.	Zinc stearate	7
4.	Magnesium carbonate	3
5.	Perfume	QS
6.	Colour	QS

Table 2.40(v)

S. No.	Ingredient	%	%
1.	Talc	60	80
2.	Zinc oxide	10	10
3.	Zinc stearate	15	5
4.	Magnesium carbonate	15	5
5.	Perfume	QS	QS
6.	Colour—ochre	QS	QS

Table 2.40(vi)

S. No.	Ingredient	%	%
1.	Talc	70	30
2.	Zinc oxide	10	20
3.	Titanium dioxide	10	5
4.	Colloidal clay	5	40
5.	Precipitated chalk	2	3
6.	Magnesium carbonate	3	2
7.	Perfume	QS	QS
8.	Colour—pink and rose	QS	QS

Table 2.40(vii)

S. No.	Ingredient	%	%
1.	Zinc stearate	5	5
2.	Talc	40	30
3.	Colloidal clay	40	10
4.	Titanium dioxide	4	5
5.	Magnesium carbonate	5	10
6.	Precipitated chalk	3	40
7.	Perfume	QS	QS
8.	Colour—lilac and lavendar	QS	QS

Table 2.40(viii)

S. No.	Ingredient	%	%
1.	Talc	20	40
2.	Colloidal clay	20	10
3.	Zinc oxide	15	15
4.	Magnesium stearate	5	10
5.	Magnesium carbonate	10	5
6.	Precipitated chalk	30	20
7.	Perfume	QS	QS
8.	Colour	QS	QS

Table 2.40(ix)

S. No.	Ingredient	%	%
1.	Talc	75	70
2.	Titanium dioxide	3	10
3.	Magnesium stearate	5	5
4.	Magnesium carbonate	10	5
5.	Rice starch	7	10
6.	Perfume	QS	QS
7.	Colour—marigold and turmeric	QS	QS

Table 2.40(x)

S. No.	Ingredient	%	%
1.	Talc	50	60
2.	Colloidal clay	12	–
3.	Titanium dioxide	10	–
4.	Magnesium stearate	3	5
5.	Magnesium carbonate	10	5
6.	Rice starch	15	30
7.	Perfume	QS	QS
8.	Colour—marigold and turmeric	QS	QS

Table 2.40(xi)

S. No.	Ingredient	%	%
1.	Talc	50	50
2.	Titanium dioxide	5	5
3.	Zinc oxide	10	10
4.	Colloidal clay	12	12
5.	Magnesium carbonate	3	6
6.	Precipitated chalk	10	10
7.	Zinc stearate	10	7
8.	Perfume	QS	QS
9.	Colour—Calendula, floral powder	QS	QS

Table 2.40(xii)

S. No.	Ingredient	%	%
1.	Talc	60	40
2.	Zinc oxide	20	30
3.	Titanium dioxide	–	8
4.	Zinc stearate	8	20
5.	Magnesium carbonate	2	–
6.	Precipitated chalk	10	2
7.	Perfume	QS	QS
8.	Colour—Marigold	QS	QS

Manufacturing

The chosen perfume is to be mixed thoroughly with a portion of magnesium carbonate in an enameled white pail or a suitable vessel. The mixture is rubbed through a hand sieve with a stiff bristle brush. When the perfume oil is thoroughly absorbed it is run through a power brush sifter until uniform distribution of the perfume is effected. Then the colour is mixed in the same way with the rest of the magnesium carbonate and chalk.

The process is continued, till no colour flakes are found, when the mixture is smeared on a paper. A sample is kept aside for matching purpose and quality control.

The colour and perfume bases are mixed with the rest of raw materials, which are blended with herbal powders. Thus, the first portion viz. colour, perfume and magnesium carbonate and chalk is mixed with the second portion, zinc stearate and zinc oxide. After thorough mixing of the two portions, the final mixture is sifted through 300 mesh. The herbal powders sometimes may be problematic, due to their fibre content. Hence, care must be taken to see that the herbal powders are pulverised into very fine particle size free from fibre.

In the process control, the final mix of the ingredients is checked with matching sample.

Fineness of particles has been described by terms like air floated, micronized and air spun depending on the process by which it is obtained. For example, in air floating, the finished powder is passed through a mill, equipped with a fan cyclone and a dust arrester to air separate the coarse particle to a predetermined height because they cannot be blown, until they are adequately fine.

A micronizer is a mill that grinds all the power particles to a desired micron size, 0.001 mm.

The air spinning process employs a method, wherein the powder is whirled around by a purified continuous air stream under great pressure. It is housed in a specially constructed cylindrical vessel. The powder particles knock against each other, at an estimated speed of over thousand miles per hour. This collision at high speed reduces the particle size. At this point the smaller particles are sucked out using the principle of centrifugal force while the larger ones remain inside, until they are divided further. Such process render uniform distribution of perfume and colour and provide greater fluffiness. Some of the manufacturers follow the practice of keeping the powder in air tight storage bins for several weeks before filling. In an another method of manufacturing, two operations are used. Firstly, the preparation of a white powder base which is perfumed and stored in airtight bins to bloom. Secondly, sufficient quantity of colour bases are made at one time for several batches and used as and when the batch is made. This process speeds up the manufacture of face powder and also help in maintaining uniformity of the batches.

Note: With all the modern micronisers and pulverisers, the desired fineness of the herbal powder is difficult to achieve due to the varieties of fibrous nature of the parts of the plants used.

Face Powders in other Forms

Cream powders, liquid powders, cake powders are quite similar to face powders in composition. The qualities that are required for face powders are the same for these products also. Cake powders are nothing but compressed powders into a compact solid tablet. Rouge is a thick coloured compact cake. Cake face powders are made by three methods:
1. Wet compression method
2. Dry compression method
3. Wet moulding

Wet Compression Method

All the ingredients of the face powder formulation are mixed thoroughly and granulated by blending this powder mix with a molten liquid and pass through a granulator. The wet granules are dried and then compressed by a compact face powder.

Dry Compression Method

All the ingredients of the face powder formulation including perfume and colour are pulverized in a ball mill and then mixed thoroughly once again till the mass becomes granular. These granules are then subjected compression. The finished cakes are dried at 60°C for one hour.

Wet Moulding

All the ingredients are made into a wet paste, rolled into lubricated nickel moulds and then allowed to dry. Dextrin or gum arabic adhesive is painted over the surface of the cakes. Then glass porcelain or metal plates are pressed down on the glued surface of the cakes. When the cakes are dried up, they adhere to the plates.

A compact should neither be too hard nor too soft. The powder should come off easily on to the puff and the cake must not get too hard and shiny. All the ingredients used are same as the ones used in a face powder. The stearates make good binders and spreading agents. The optimum maximum percentage of talc in cakes is 50–60%. The viscosity or binding solutions should be standardized and should be uniform throughout the batches. In general the binding materials are made from gum karaya, acacia, quince seeds, rosin, irish moss. Sometimes, lanolin dissolved in ether is used. All these binding solutions are preserved with safe preservatives.

Face Powder Compact

Table 2.41

S. No.	Solutions	Parts
1.	Gum tragacanth	20
2.	Quince seed mucilage	10
3.	Gelatin mucilage	10
4.	Rosin tincture	
5.	Water	60
6.	Preservative (methyl p-hydroxybenzoate)	

In all the above mentioned formulae, the base composition is given, the choice of colour and perfume is left to the formulator.

Table 2.42

Base powder formula		
S. No.	Ingredient	%
1.	Talc (300 mesh)	50
2.	Zinc oxide	20
3.	Zinc stearate	6
4.	Rice starch	10
5.	Magnesium carbonate	4
6.	Colloidal clay	10
7.	Colour	QS
8.	Perfume	QS
9.	Herbal powder mix	QS

Manufacturing

All the ingredients of the base formula are pulverised through a ball mill. After pulverizing the base powders including the herbal powder is moistened, with a sufficient quantity of binding solution till the powder becomes granular and suitable to the type of process that is going to be selected for compression into cake.

Table 2.43(i)

S. No.	Ingredient	%
	Base powder formula	
1.	Talc	70
2.	Zinc oxide	15
3.	Gum mucilage	7
5.	Perfume	8
6.	Colour	QS

Table 2.43(ii)

S. No.	Ingredient	%
	Base	
1.	Kaolin	40
2.	Talc	40
3.	Magnesium carbonate	10
4.	Rice starch	10
5.	Perfume	QS
6.	Anhydrous lanolin in ether	QS

All the powdered materials are mixed thoroughly in a mixer together with the colour till the mass becomes granular with lanolin solution.

Process Technology

The formulae designed should be standardized with optimum percentages and reproducible results should be obtainable. All the unit operations, like mixing and drying and degree of fineness of powders must be kept uniform. Generally cake make up exclusively leaves a flat, smooth and lasting finish on the skin. It also covers minor blemishes.

The consumer should feel comfortable after the application of powder on the skin. A well formulated cake should come out easily with a moistened tissue or sponge as an emulsion and cover the skin uniformly. The film produced on the skin should not draw the skin by drying out quickly, remain on the skin throughout the day, repel moisture caused by perspiration and be easily removed by washing with water or soap water.

The raw materials that can contribute to the above properties are given below:

Titanium dioxide and zinc oxide	–	Covering and masking properties to the cake.
Kaolin and colloidal clay	–	Help as binders in compressing but excessive usage is not advised as it may cause too much absorption of water, causing piling up of the film.
Chalk	–	Regulates easy brushing off or blending with skin.
Talc	–	Stable filler, but if used in excess shine will be imparted.

Note: Care must be taken in combining these ingredients judiciously with the clay to get the desired effect and performance.

Pigments selected should not bleed during perspiration. Normally water insoluble lakes and mineral pigments are preferred. Vegetable oils will provide the desired oilyness. As vegetable oils are prone to turn rancid, anti-oxidants are to be included in the oils. The manufacturing of make up cakes differs when compared to compacts. First the powders are mixed. The water–oil emulsion and humectants are subsequently added and the mixture is passed through a roller mixer for better homogenicity. The resultant paste is then granulated and pressed into cakes.

Liquid Powders

These are used for evening wear to counter the glare of electric lights. They are applied to face, neck and arms and serve to blend the colours of the skin exposed only in the evening dress due to their high opacity.

All the above ingredients are stirred into the oil solution of magnesium oleate and allowed to stand overnight. Care must be taken to ensure that the final product does not become too tacky and dries off reasonably quickly.

Table 2.44(i)

S. No.	Herbal liquid powders formula Ingredient	%
1.	Colloidal clay	10
2.	Titanium dioxide	18
3.	Glycerin	2
4.	Water	70
5.	Perfume	QS
6.	Colour	QS

Table 2.44(ii)

S. No.	Ingredient	%
1.	Colloidal clay	10
2.	Precipitated chalk	7
3.	Zinc oxide	10
4.	Glycerin	3
5.	Alcohol	7
6.	Floral water and powder mix	63

Table 2.44(iii)

S. No.	Ingredient	%
1.	Talc	10
2.	Colloidal clay	7
3.	Glycerin	10
4.	Kewda floral dust	3
5.	Water	60
6.	Alcohol	10

Table 2.44(iv)

S. No.	Ingredient	%
1.	Colloidal zinc oxide	12
2.	Precipitated chalk	5
3.	Colloidal clay	5
4.	Zinc stearate	2
5.	Glycerin	3
6.	Elangi mimosa floral dust	3
7.	Water	70

Table 2.44(v)

S. No.	Ingredient	%
1.	Titanium dioxide	5
2.	Precipitated chalk	5
3.	Colloidal clay	15
4.	Glycerin	5
5.	Water and powder	70

Table 2.44(vi)

S. No.	Ingredient	%
1.	Colloidal zinc oxide	10
2.	Colloidal clay	5
3.	Precipitated chalk heavy	6
4.	Glycerin	5
5.	Night queen	10
6.	Floral water	64

Table 2.44(vii)

S. No.	Ingredient	%
1.	Heavy mineral oil	60
2.	Magnesium oleate	27
3.	Titanium dioxide	5
4.	Light chalk	5
5.	Perfume	QS
6.	Red-iron oxide	1
7.	Ochre liquid	1
8.	Nyctanthes powder flowers	1

Manufacturing

All the powdered ingredients and colour are mixed including herbal/floral powder in a powder mixer. The liquid ingredients are blended in another tank, with an agitator. The powders are slowly drawn into the blended liquid with agitation. After thorough mixing, the whole mass is slowed to settle for half an hour. Then it is subjected for filling with the stirrer in motion to ensure uniform mixing.

Table 2.45

Cream powder		
S. No.	Ingredient	%
1.	Vanishing cream base	60
2.	Talc	20
3.	Titanium dioxide	10
4.	Herbal powder	10
5.	Perfume—natural colon	QS

Mix all the above ingredients including colour and perfume and pass through a roller mill.

Table 2.46(i)

S. No.	Cream powder base	
	Ingredient	%
1.	Glyceryl monostearate	8
2.	Glycerin	12
3.	Heavy mineral oil	10
4.	Spermaceti	10
5.	Stearic acid	5
6.	Potassium hydroxide	0.15
7.	Water	50
8.	Titanium dioxide	5
9.	Perfume	QS

Table 2.46(ii)

S. No.	Ingredient	%
1.	Glycerin	20
2.	Stearic acid	10
3.	White face powder	42
4.	Distilled water	28
5.	Potassium hydroxide (I.P.)	1
6.	Perfume	QS

Make a solution of potassium hydroxide in water and add this to molten stearic acid. After the saponification is over, heat the glycerin and add the face powder, colour and mix till uniform mixing of both liquid and solid phases is obtained. Then add the saponified mass, perfume and mix again. Then pass the product through an ointment mill to ensure smoothness and uniformity of colour distribution.

Quality Control

Degree of fineness and colour blending should be uniform. Colours should not bleed out when applied on the face.

Evaluation

1. Should cover the face, maximum area with minimum quantity.
2. Colour blending should be uniform
3. Perfume should be mild pleasant, soothing, lingering and with uniform intensity, form the date of manufacturing till the last day of shelf life.
4. Minimum number of applications on the face should help it look fresh without shine.

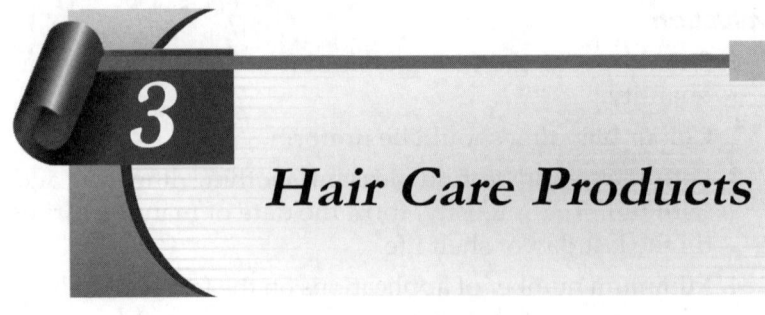

3

Hair Care Products

Hair lends beauty to the face more so in the case of women. Hair care products are developed with this criterion as the starting point. The major requirement of classification of hair care products is to make the hair look manageable and promote healthy growth.

The products that are aimed at this are broadly:

1. **Hair grooming:** Hair oils, pomades, brilliantines for grooming, manageability, maintenance for any desired hair dressing.
2. **Hair tonics:** For prevention of hair loss and promotion of hair growth.
3. **Hair creams:** For the convenience and comfort in application. Hair creams can be called as an extension of hair oils.
4. **Conditioning:** Shampoos, leave-on conditions.
5. **Hair setting lotions:** To keep the hair dressing intact.
6. **Hair dyes:** In order to colour the hair and mask the grey hair, dyes are used.
7. **Miscellaneous:** Anti-lice, antidandruff, cause health to the hair. Hair "therapeutics."

- Hair oils
- Hair tonics
- Hair creams
- Hair setting lotions
- Hair dyes
- Shampoos
- Miscellaneous

Table 3.1: Plants used in hair care products

S. No.	Herbs	Parts used	Property
1.	Acacia concinna (Fig. 3.1)	Pods	Cleansing
2.	Albizzia amara (Fig. 3.2)	Leaves	Cleansing
3.	Datura metel (Fig. 3.3)	Leaves	Antidandruff
4.	Aloe barbadensis (Fig. 3.4)	Leaves	Conditioner
5.	Alternanthera sessilis (Fig. 3.5)	Leaves	Cooling, hair colouring
6.	Amaranthus spinosus (Fig. 3.6)	Leaves	Hair colouring
7.	Annona squamosa (Fig. 3.7)	Leaves, seeds	Anti-lice
8.	Camellia sinensis (Fig. 3.8)	Flowers	Flavouring
9.	Centella asiatica (Fig. 3.9)	Leaves	Cooling and memory
10.	Citrus limon (Fig. 3.10)	Leaves, fruit rind	Refreshing, flavouring
11.	Coffea arabica (Fig. 3.11)	Seeds	Hair colouring
12.	Eclipta alba (Fig. 3.12)	Leaves	Hair growth promoter
13.	Emblica officinalis (Fig. 3.13)	Fruits	Colouring and pH adjusting
14.	Hibiscus rosa sinensis (Fig. 3.14)	Flowers	Hair growth promoter
15.	Indigofera tinctoria (Fig. 3.15)	Leaves	Hair colouring
16.	Lawsonia inermis (Fig. 3.16)	Leaves	Hair colouring
17.	Mirabilis jalapa (Fig. 3.17)	Roots	Hair growth promoter
18.	Muraya koenigii (Fig. 3.18)	Leaves	Hair colouring
19.	Musa acuminata—flower (Fig. 3.19)	Flowers	Hair colouring, cooling
20.	Musa acuminata—root (Fig. 3.20)	Roots	Hair colouring, cooling
21.	Nardostachys jatamansi (Fig. 3.21)	Roots	Hair growth promoter
22.	Quercus infectoria (Fig. 3.22)	Galls	Hair colouring
23.	Rosmarinus officinalis (Fig. 3.23)	Entire plant	Hair growth promoter
24.	Salvia officinalis (Fig. 3.24)	Leaves	Hair colouring
25.	Sapindus mukorossi (Fig. 3.25)	Fruits	Cleansing
26.	Sesamum indicum (Fig. 3.26)	Seed oil	Hair growth promoter
27.	Terminalia chebula (Fig. 3.27)	Fruits	Mordant in colour
28.	Trigonella foenum-graecum (Fig. 3.28)	Seeds	Viscosity builder, conditioner
29.	Urtica dioica (Fig. 3.29)	Leaves	Antidandruff

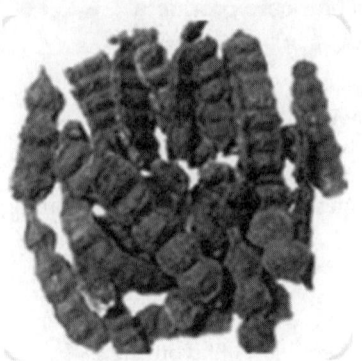

Fig. 3.1: *Acacia concinna*

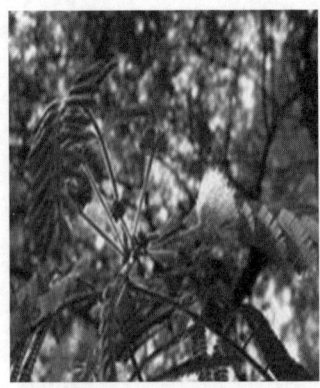

Fig. 3.2: *Albizzia amara*

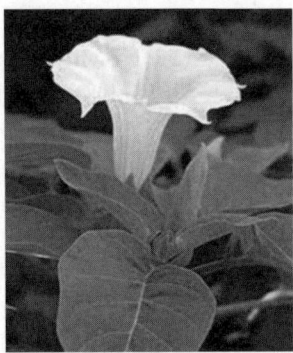

Fig. 3.3: *Datura metel*

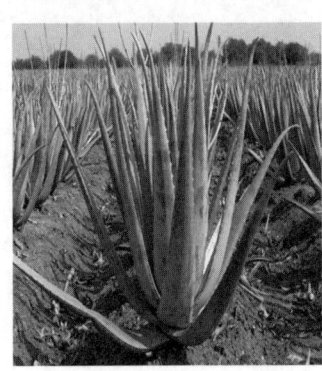

Fig. 3.4: *Aloe barbadensis*

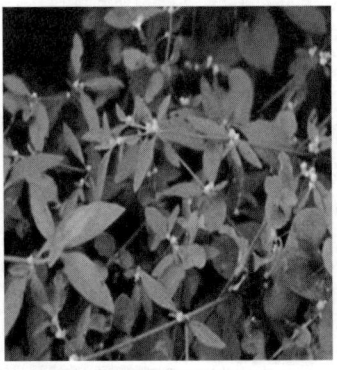

Fig. 3.5: *Alternanthera sessilis*

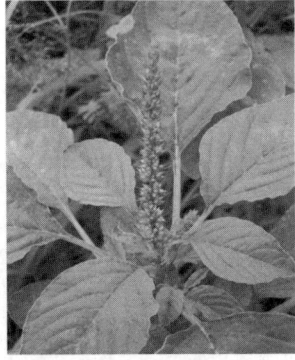

Fig. 3.6: *Amaranthus spinosus*

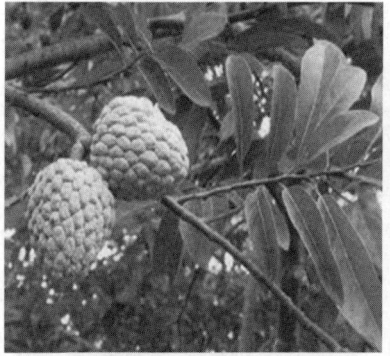

Fig. 3.7: *Annona squamosa*

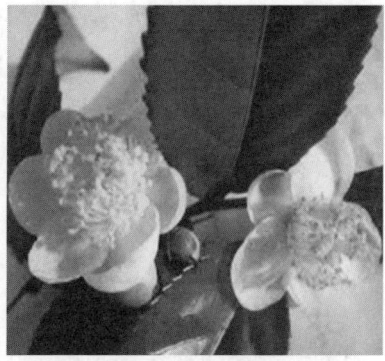

Fig. 3.8: *Camellia sinensis*

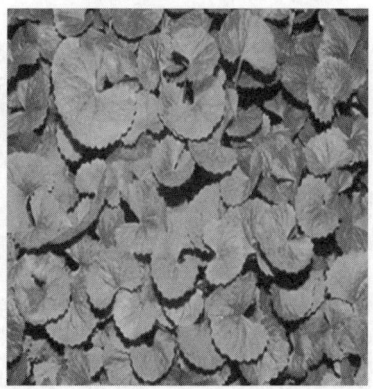

Fig. 3.9: *Centella asiatica*

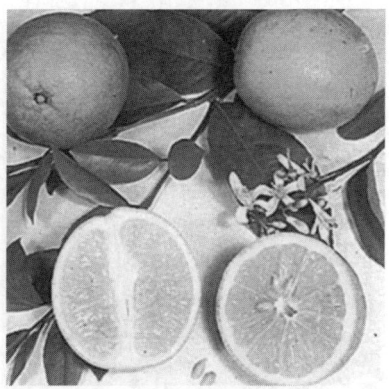

Fig. 3.10: *Citrus limon*

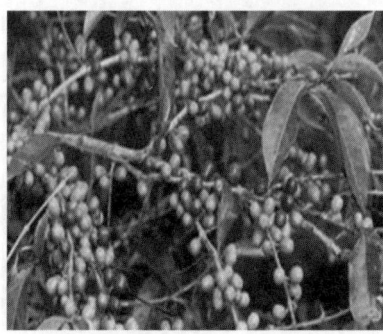

Fig. 3.11: *Coffea arabica*

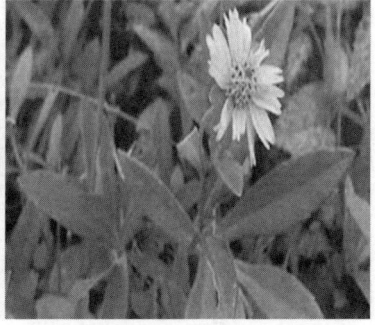

Fig. 3.12: *Eclipta alba*

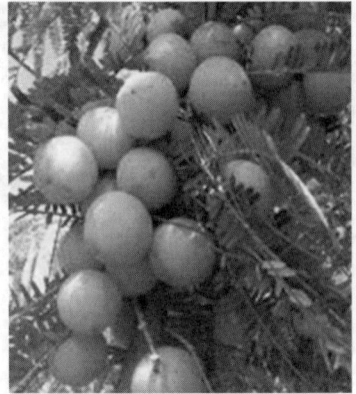

Fig. 3.13: *Emblica officinalis*

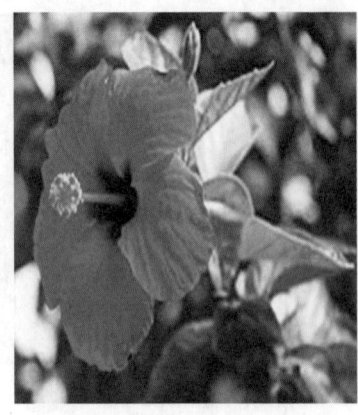

Fig. 3.14: *Hibiscus rosa sinensis*

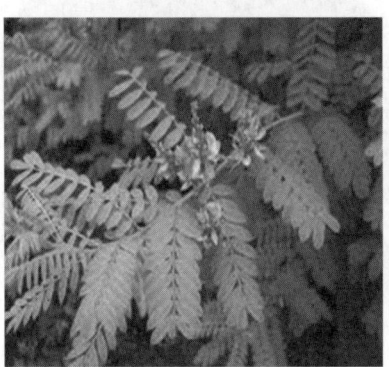

Fig. 3.15: *Indigofera tinctoria*

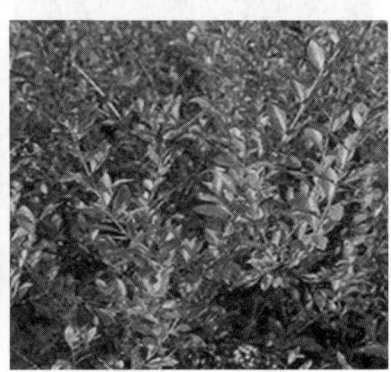

Fig. 3.16: *Lawsonia inermis*

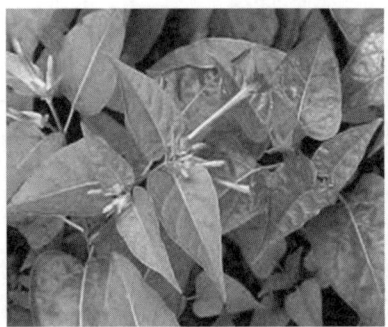

Fig. 3.17: *Mirabilis jalapa*

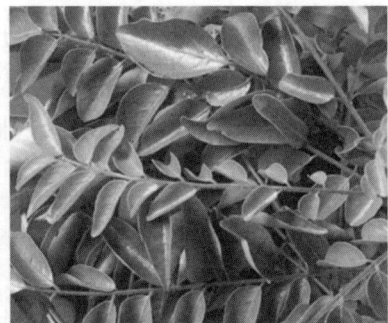

Fig. 3.18: *Muraya koenigii*

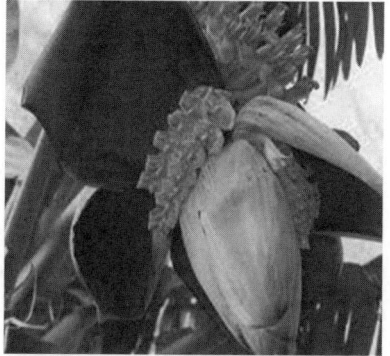

Fig. 3.19: *Musa acuminata*—flower

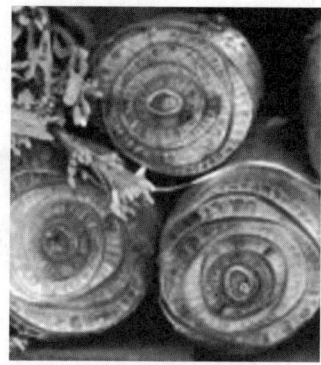

Fig. 3.20: *Musa acuminata*—root

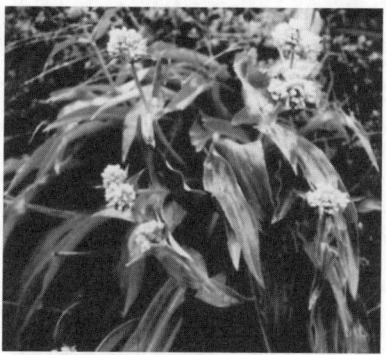

Fig. 3.21: *Nardostachys jatamansi*

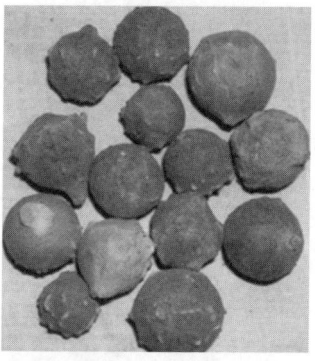

Fig. 3.22: *Quercus infectoria*

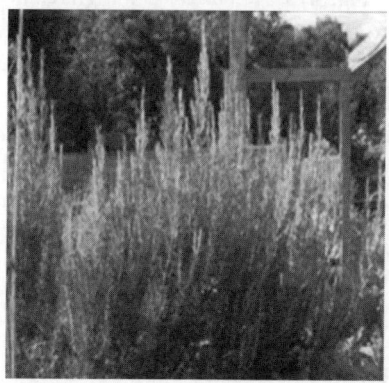

Fig. 3.23: *Rosmarinus officinalis*

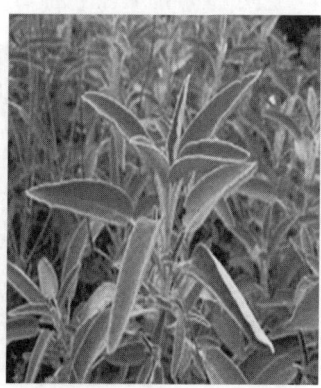

Fig. 3.24: *Salvia officinalis*

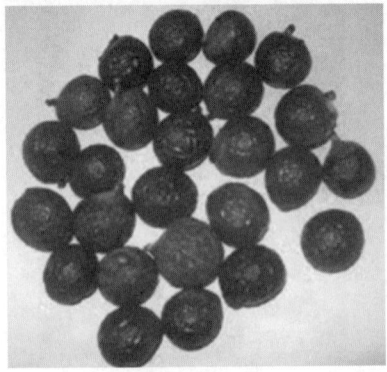

Fig. 3.25: *Sapindus mukorossi*

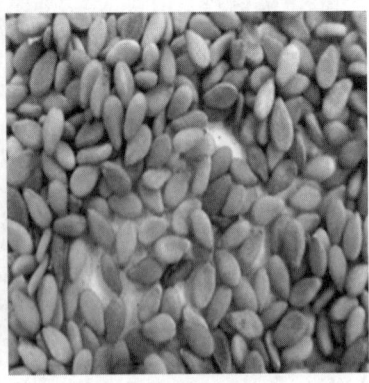

Fig. 3.26. *Sesamum indicum*

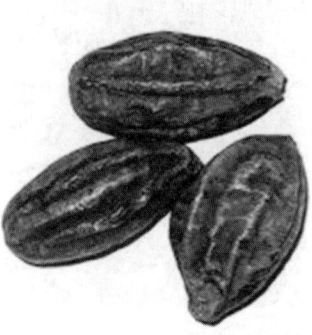

Fig. 3.27: *Terminalia chebula*

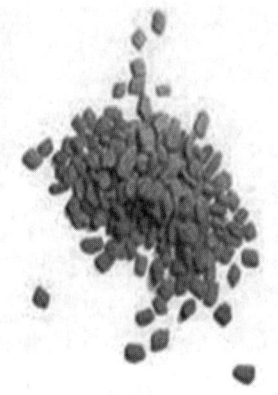

Fig. 3.28: *Trigonella foenum-graecum*

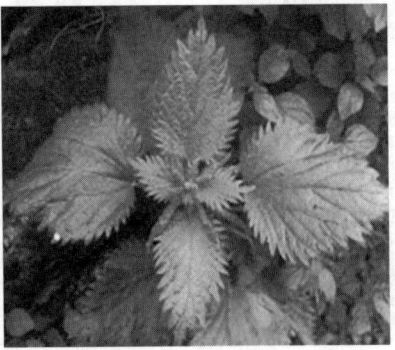

Fig. 3.29: *Urtica dioica*

HAIR OILS

A healthy being reflects his/her health through thick glossy, shiny hair. Hair oils are external preparations mostly used for manageability of the hair and in hair dressing. However, some of the hair oils are enriched for hair growth and prevention of hair fall. Plants that are useful for such a purpose are *Lawsonia inermis, Nardostachys jatamansi, Hibiscus rosa sinensis* flowers, and *Rosemaria officinalis* oil. At one time, long, strong and thick hair was desirable and popular because these qualities were seen as beauty enhancers.

Nowadays short and flying hair is the order of the day. However, for thick and glossy hair, hair oils are helpful, through massage, in strengthening the hair roots and making them strong which helps in preventing hair loss and promoting hair growth. In India, coconut oil is the main vehicle or base used for making hair oils. Ayurvedic hair oils are made out of gingelly oil and a mixture of gingelly oil (til oil) and coconut oil with herbs that promote growth of the hair and prevent falling or loss of hair.

Formulations

Table 3.2

Base			Herbal extracts mix		
S. No.	*Ingredient*	*%*	*S. No.*	*Ingredient*	*Parts*
1.	Coconut oil	80	1.	*Lawsonia inermis*	10
2.	Gingelly oil	10	2.	*Musa acuminata*—root juice	10
3.	Sunflower oil	3			
4.	Herbal extract mix	7	3.	*Eclipta alba*	8
5.	Perfume	QS	4.	*Hibiscus rosa sinensis* flower	8
			5.	*Centella asiatica*	3
			6.	*Emblica officinalis*	10
			7.	*Citrus limon*—juice	6
			8.	*Nardostachys jatamansi*—root	3
			9.	*Rosmarinus officinalis*—oil	2

Table 3.3

Base			Herbal extracts mix		
S. No.	Ingredient	%	S. No.	Ingredient	Parts
1.	Coconut oil	80	1.	Eclipta alba	10
2.	Almond oil	10	2.	Emblica officinalis	10
3.	Sunflower oil	10	3.	Citrus limon	10

Table 3.4

Base			Herbal extracts mix		
S. No.	Ingredient	%	S. No.	Ingredient	Parts
1.	Til oil	70	1.	Centella asiatica	10
2.	Almond oil	10	2.	Emblica officinalis	10
3.	Apricot oil	10	3.	Hibiscus rosa sinensis	10
4.	Sunflower oil	10	4.	Amarantus census	10
			5.	Musa acuminata—root	10

Manufacturing

All the plant ingredients (coarse powders) are extracted with water in the ratio 1:5 and boiled in the base oil till clear.

Quality Control

The hair oil is to be checked for the following parameters to maintain quality:

1. Colour
2. Refractive index
3. Specific gravity
4. Clarity

Quality Control Assurance

All the raw materials (herbs) are to be of pharmacopoeial grade with reproducibility in quality and purity.

Packing and Storage

Unit packs can be made in either HDP or PVC containers.

Evaluation

Absorption, penetration into scalp, prevention of hair fall, promoting manageability, hair grooming.

HAIR TONICS

Hair products which promote hair growth, arrest hair fall and strengthen hair roots are hair tonics.

Formulations
Table 3.5

Base			Herbal extracts mix		
S. No.	Ingredient	%	S. No.	Ingredient	Parts
1.	Coconut oil	70	1.	Nardostachys jatamansi	8
2.	Almond oil	20	2.	Eclipta alba	5
3.	Castor oil	10	3.	Mirabilis jalapa	10
			4.	Rosmarinus officinalis—oil	2

Table 3.6

Base			Herbal extracts mix		
S. No.	Ingredient	%	S. No.	Ingredient	Parts
1.	Coconut oil	70	1.	Nardostachys jatamansi	8
2.	Almond oil	20	2.	Eclipta alba	5
3.	Til oil	10	3.	Rosmarinus officinalis–oil	2

Table 3.7

Base			Herbal extracts mix		
S. No.	Ingredient	%	S. No.	Ingredient	Parts
1.	Coconut oil	80	1.	Emblica officinalis	10
2.	Almond oil	10	2.	Centella asiatica	10
3.	Castor oil	5	3.	Musa acuminata—root	10
4.	Sunflower oil	5	4.	Hibiscus rosa sinensis	10
			5.	Amarantus census	10

Manufacturing

All the plant ingredients (coarse powders) are extracted with water in the ratio 1:5 and boiled in the base oil till clear.

Quality Control

The separated oil phase from the extracts is to be checked for the following parameters:

1. Colour
2. Viscosity
3. Refractive index
4. Specific gravity.

Packing and Storage

Unit packs can be made in either HDP or PVC containers.

Evaluation

Clear and transparent oil with non-greasy feeling, prevention of hair loss and promotion of hair growth.

HAIR CREAMS

Herbal hair oils processed into creams are also very useful as dressing preparations in hair grooming. The product is consumer friendly and serves the purpose of hair oil without its greasiness. Basically these creams are o/w type emulsions.

Formulations

Table 3.8

S. No.	Ingredient	%
1.	Herbal hair oil	30
2.	Triethanolamine	10
3.	Glycerin	10
4.	Water	45
5.	Borax	5
6.	Hina perfume	QS

Manufacturing

Both oil and water phases are heated up to 70°C and then stirred for half an hour before they are fed into a colloid mill. When the temperature falls down to 50°C , perfume and colour are added and milled once again before emptied into the SS storage vessel.

Table 3.9(i)

S. No.	Ingredient	%
1.	Beeswax	7
2.	Emulsifying wax	3
3.	Herbal hair oil	33
4.	Water	54
5.	Borax	2
6.	Glycerol monostearate (GMS)	1
7.	Perfume	QS

Manufacturing

Oil and waxes or the oily phase are heated to 70°C and then water and borax are mixed and heated up to 72°C. Water is added to oil phase and both the phases are mixed with constant stirring, allowed to settle till the mix congeals at 45°C into a uniform solid mass.

Table 3.9(ii)

S. No.	Ingredient	%
1.	Herbal hair oil	60
2.	Almond oil	5
3.	Castor oil	25
4.	Ethyl alcohol	10
5.	Colour	QS
6.	Perfume	QS

Table 3.9(iii)

S. No.	Ingredient	%
1.	Herbal hair oil	50
2.	Ethyl myristate	5
3.	Beeswax	3
4.	Stearic acid	2
5.	Lanolin	2
6.	Water	38
7.	Colour	QS
8.	Perfume	QS

Table 3.9(iv)

S. No.	Ingredient	%
1.	Herbal hair oil	49.5
2.	Lanolin	2
3.	Beeswax	18
4.	Magnesium sulphate	0.1
5.	Sodium hydroxide	0.4
6.	Water	30
7.	Colour	QS
8.	Perfume	QS

Table 3.9(v)

S. No.	Ingredient	%
1.	Herbal hair oil	45
2.	Wax	3
3.	Beeswax	3
4.	Stearic acid	3
5.	Spermaceti	3
6.	Emulsifying wax	3
7.	Water	40
8.	Colour	QS
9.	Perfume	QS

Table 3.9(vi)

S. No.	Ingredient	%
1.	Herbal hair oil	50
2.	Cetyl alcohol	3
3.	Beeswax	5
4.	Stearic acid	2
5.	Water	40
6.	Colour	QS
7.	Perfume	QS

Manufacturing

All these materials are heated together to 55°C and cooled to room temperature before bottling. These creams will add sheen to the hair and help in grooming it.

Quality Control

Specific gravity, viscosity (80 cps), spreadability.

Quality Control Assurance

All the raw materials/ingredients used in manufacturing should be of reproducible quality and purity.

Packing and Storage

When the mass congeals to 45°C, the cream is subjected to filling in tubes, glass or plastic containers and stored away from heat and light.

Evaluation

The final product should be transparent or even translucent and should help in manageability in hair grooming.

High Glossy Hair Emulsions

Absorption Base Formula

Table 3.10(i)

S. No.	Ingredient	%
1.	Herbal hair oil	47
2.	Beeswax	4
3.	Borax	3
4.	Stearic acid	1
5.	Lime water	45
6.	Perfume	QS

Table 3.10(ii)

S. No.	Ingredient	%
1.	Absorption base	6
2.	Beeswax	2
3.	Herbal hair oil	57
4.	Glycerol	2
5.	Triethanolamine	3
6.	Water	30
7.	Perfume	QS

Table 3.10(iii)

S. No.	Ingredient	%
1.	Absorption base	6
2.	Beeswax	2
3.	Herbal hair oil	58
4.	Glycerol	1
5.	Triethanolamine	3
6.	Water	30
7.	Perfume	QS

Manufacturing

Beeswax in the oil phase is melted and poured into triethanol-amine and water. The oil phase is heated up to 75°C and the water phase up to 70°C before mixing. The resultant mixture is homogenized.

Hair Dressing Emulsions

Table 3.11

S. No.	Ingredient	%
1.	Herbal hair oil	45
2.	Beeswax	3
3.	Soft paraffin	8
4.	Absorption base	7
5.	Water	37

Alcoholic Extract of the Following Herbs

Table 3.12

S. No.	Ingredient	%
1.	Herbal hair oil	57
2	*Musa acuminate* flower extract	3
3.	*Trigonella foenum-graecum* extract	2
4.	*Aloe barbadensis* extract	2
5.	Absorption base	6
6.	Water	30

Manufacturing

The herbs extract, water and absorption base are warmed, to 65°C stirred for 1 hour and allowed to cool. It is kept aside for 24 hours under observation.

Quality Control

The mixture should be uniform, i.e. without separating into the two phases.

Packing and Storage

Packed in plastic bottles and stored away from light and heat.

Evaluation

On application to hair, the hair should appear glossy and non-greasy, easily washable.

HAIR SETTING LOTIONS IN SPRAY PACKING

These are mainly for keeping the position of the hair on the scalp intact. Usually polymeric substances are used. But natural herbal extracts can be used as substitutes.

Table 3.13

S. No.	Ingredient	%
1.	Herbal hair oil	54
2.	Paraffin	8
3.	Beeswax	3
4.	Ceralan	5
5.	Water	30

Table 3.14

Herbal extracts mix		
S. No.	Ingredient	%
1.	*Musa acuminata* flower	3
2.	*Trigonella foenum-graecum*	2
3.	*Aloe barbadensis*	1
4.	Gum karaya	1
5.	Absorption base	5
6.	Water	88
7.	Perfume	QS
8.	Colour	QS

Manufacturing

Aqueous extracts of the plants in aqueous phase are mixed with water and this is emulsified with 6% absorption base and packed in spray packs.

Quality Control

For spray covering area and keeping the hair intact from flying.

Packing and Storage

Packed in spray containers and stored away from light and heat.

Evaluation

After spraying on the hair, the hair should be in position. Hair sheen should be enhanced.

HAIR DYES

Hair dyes are used to hide grey hair. Today there are a number of hair dyes that have found way into the market. The most popular chemical hair dye is paraphenylene diamine (PPD). But it carries with it a heavy burden of harmful synthetic/side effects. *Lawsonia inermis* and *Indigofera tinctoria* present a safer and natural alternative.

Herbal hair dyes originated in Persia. Men coloured their grey beard and women their hair with henna and *Indigofera tinctoria*. But today many shades of hair dyes/colours are available in the shelf.

Natural Hair Dyes

1. *Lawsonia inermis*
2. Chamomile
3. *Indigofera tinctoria*
4. *Salvia officinalis*

A typical grey hair blackening natural plant dye.

Formulations

Table 3.15

S. No.	Ingredient	%
1.	Lawsonia inermis—powder	75
2.	Indigofera tinctoria	20
3.	Quercus infectoria—powder	5

Extract of these powders will give a brownish black colour.

Table 3.16

S. No.	Ingredient	%
1.	Lawsonia inermis—leaf powder	50
2.	Mango seed	20
3.	Hibiscus rosa sinensis	10
4.	Musa acuminata—root	10
5.	Eclipta alba	10

Table 3.17

S. No.	Ingredient	%
1.	Lawsonia inermis—powder	60
2.	Indigofera tinctoria	25
3.	Terminalia chebula	5
4.	Musa acuminata—root	5
5.	Eclipta alba powder	5

Manufacturing

All the powders are mixed in water to make a paste and applied with a brush on the hair after washing. Keep it for an hour and shampoo it to enhance the shade. Herbal amla hair oil will help in giving a darker shade when applied after washing or rinsing the hair with shampoo and water.

Table 3.18

S. No.	Ingredient	%
1.	*Lawsonia inermis*	60
2.	*Indigofera tinctoria*—leaves powder	10
3.	Coffee extract	5
4.	*Eclipta alba*—powder	15
5.	*Quercus infectoria*—powder	5
6.	*Trigonella foenum-graecum*	5

Manufacturing

All are mixed and made into a paste before applying on the hair (preferably washed and wet). Keep it for one hour, shampoo the hair and rinse with water. The herbal hair oil preferably amla hair oil, on application over the dyed hair will enhance the blackish brown colour on the grey hair.

Table 3.19

S. No.	Ingredient	%
1.	*Lawsonia inermis*—powder	70
2.	*Indigofera tinctoria*	10
3.	*Terminalia chebula*—powder	7
4.	*Salvia officinalis* (sage)	13

All powders are mixed with water into a paste.

Table 3.20

S. No.	Ingredient	%
1.	*Acacia catechu*	10
2.	Wallnut shell powder	4
3.	*Quercus infectoria*	6
4.	*Lawsonia alba*	60
5.	*Hibiscus rosa sinensis*	10
6.	*Salvia officinalis*	10

Table 3.21

S. No.	Ingredient	%
1.	*Lawsonia inermis* powder	60
2.	Mango seed—powder	20
3.	*Eclipta alba*	5
4.	*Terminalia chebula*	15

In acidic pH dark brown shade.

Table 3.22

S. No.	Ingredient	%
1.	Rhubarb	10
2.	*Lawsonia inermis*	75
3.	*Salvia officinalis*	10
4.	Potassium hydroxide	5

Manufacturing

All the plants are powdered and extracted and then soaked in 5% alkaline solution. The varieties of herbal dyes are commercially not very viable due to lack of depth in the colour and instability of the powders which are very vulnerable to oxidation. Hence, these are less widely recommended, although they are safe.

Quality Control

Wetting capacity, spreadabilitly, mordancy to the hair.

Packing and Storage

Packed in unit packs of single application say 50 g in air tight polythene bags placed in an outer silver foil pouch and stored away from light and heat.

Evaluation

Hair should not get decolourised. Frequency of application should be minimum, bimonthly.

HERBAL SHAMPOO

The word shampoo is a Hindustani word meaning squeezing. It is meant for cleaning the hair and scalp from grease, dirt and dust. The base is usually made out of mild detergents, e.g. alkyl sulfates and olefin sulphate.

Shampoos with herbal cleansing agents are strictly herbal shampoos rather than synthetic detergent base mixed with herbal extracts. Simply because they contain herbal extracts, they cannot be strictly categorized as herbal shampoos. But the formulations with natural foaming agents, like saponins is tricky as these are very vulnerable to hydrolysis and instability. Hence, usually a safe and mild base is selected in formulation, which is a carrier of herbal extracts that are beneficial for scalp and hair.

Ingredients of a Shampoo

1. Detergents
2. Thickeners and foam stabilizers
3. Opacifiers and pearlisers
4. Conditioners
5. Other additives
6. Diluents
7. Foaming agents

Preservatives of a Shampoo

1. Diazolidinyl
2. Methylchloroisothiazolinone
3. Methylisothiazolinone
4. Sodium iodate

Additives

1. Opacifying agents
2. Stearyl alcohol
3. Cetyl alcohol
4. Behenic acid

Foam Builders

Thickening agents—herbal thickening agents like fenugreek mucilage 1–3% can also be considered.

Foam stabilizers—preservatives cetrimide, parabens, bronidiol.

Opacifying agents—CDEA (cocodiethanolamide), CMEA (cocomonoethanolamide)

Pearling agents—EGMS (Ethylene glycol monostearate)

Properties of Ideal Shampoo

1. It should not decolorize the natural colour of the hair.
2. It should cleanse the hair from grease, dust debris, etc.
3. It should not alter the natural conditioning of hair, to keep it soft.
4. It should give sufficient foam to cleanse and remove the dirt from the hair.
5. It should be compatible with hard and soft water.
6. It should not irritate mucous membrane, skin or scalp.

There can be more than one property in a single ingredient, e.g. fenugreek extract helps in conditioning, thickening and foam stabilizing.

Most of the commercial herbal shampoos are detergent based with herbal extracts. It is because the natural saponins from either *Sapindus* or *Acacia concinna* are very vulnerable to hydrolysis and they have a very short shelf life. The cost of improving the stability of these saponins is not economical, but only of academic interest.

Pearlisers

This is just to enhance the aesthetic appeal.

Formulations

Table 3.23

Base			Herbal extracts mix		
S. No.	Ingredient	%	S. No.	Ingredient	Parts
1.	Mild surfactant	55	1.	Eclipta alba	4
2.	Cocamidopropyl betaine	14	2.	Musa acuminata—root	3
3.	Polyethylene glycol	25	3.	Centella asiatica	3
4.	Herbal extract mix	6	4.	Aloe barbadensis	2
5.	Preservatives	QS	5.	Trigonella foenum-graecum	1
6.	Colour	QS			

Table 3.24

Base			Herbal extracts mix		
S. No.	Ingredient	%	S. No.	Ingredient	Parts
1.	Mild detergent—SLES	47	1.	Lawsonia inermis	5
2.	Cocamidopropyl betaine	15	2.	Mirabilis jalapa	5
3.	Distearate	5	3.	Muraya koenigii	3
4.	Herbs extract mix	8			
5.	Foaming agent miranol	5			
6.	Sorbitan mono-oleate glycol	20			
7.	Perfume	QS			
8.	Preservatives	QS			
9.	Colour	QS			

Vegetable Oil Shampoo

Table 3.25

Base			Herbal extracts mix		
S. No.	Ingredient	%	S. No.	Ingredient	Parts
1.	Coconut oil	8	1.	Hibiscus rosa sinensis	5
2.	Olive oil	6	2.	Alternanthera sessilis	2
3.	Potassium hydroxide	3			
4.	Sodium hydroxide	3			
5.	Water	70			
6.	Herbal extract mix	10			
7.	Perfume	QS			
8.	Preservatives	QS			
9.	Colour	QS			

Herbal Shampoo

Table 3.26

Base			Herbal extracts mix		
S. No.	Ingredient	%	S. No.	Ingredient	Parts
1.	Ritha extract	5	1.	Musa acuminata— root	3
2.	Ammonium carbonate	1	2.	Aloe barbadensis	3
3.	Detergent—SLES	40	3.	Emblica officinalis	2
4.	Water	20			
5.	Propylene glycol	30			
6.	Polyethylene glycol	4			
7.	Preservatives	QS			
8.	Perfume	QS			

Table 3.27

Base			Herbal extracts mix		
S. No.	Ingredient	%	S. No.	Ingredient	Parts
1.	Non-ionic detergents	15	1.	Aloe barbadensis	2
2.	Glycerol	3	2.	Eclipta alba	3
3.	Igepal	2			
4.	Sodium hexyl sulfo-acetate	6			
5.	Sodium citrate	2			
6.	Gum karaya	1			
7.	Herbal extract mix	6			
8.	Water	65			

Manufacturing

All the ingredients are mixed and stirred for half an hour. Lastly, preservatives, colour and perfume are also mixed and stirred once again for uniform mixing and kept aside overnight to settle before filling.

Quality Control and Evaluation

Shampoos should be tested for quantity and quality of the foam as well as for the rapidity of its formation. This is done initially by checking the shampoo on the hands which must be absolutely clean since otherwise the first washing will yield less foam. For comparative testing, the shampoo should be measured in a 1 ml beaker. The test is also useful for checking the smoothness of the foam, its density (light or heavy), after-feel and odor. When all these factors are satisfactory, the final test is on the hair.

For routine quality control, the shampoo should always be checked for its viscosity and pH. Viscosity should not be below 1000 centipoise to minimize running off. Medium viscosity shampoos have viscosities of about 2000 centipoise, and 3000 centipoise or above for high viscosity.

Artificial hair is used to cleanse and the height of foam is measured, compared with general ingredients of a shampoo.

Packing and Storage

Packed in containers of 100 ml, 200 ml and 500 ml in pet transparent bottles and stored away from light and heat.

Powder Shampoos

A mix of herbal powders exhibiting conditioning and cleansing propreties.

Table 3.28

S. No.	Ingredient	%
1.	Albizzia amara—leaf powder	20
2.	Sapindus mukorossi—powder	25
3.	Acacia concinna—pods powder	25
4.	Green gram powder	20
5.	Rice powder	5
6.	Trigonella foenum-graecum—seeds powder	5

Arapu leaf powder mixed with rice flour and green gram dal is a useful conditioning powder shampoo. All these are milled into powder, applied to hair with little water as a paste. It gives a very mild foam when applied on the hair but cleanses and conditions the hair.

Table 3.29

S. No.	Ingredient	%
1.	*Sapindus mukorossi*—fruit powder	70
2.	*Hibiscus rosa sinensis*—leaf powder	10
3.	*Trigonella foenum-graecum*—powder	10
4.	Green gram powder	10

Manufacturing

All the above ingredients are milled and sieved through 80–100 mesh.

Quality Control

The powder should easily mix with and wash off the hair easily. It should not clog and drain.

Packing and Storage

Packed in units of 100 g, 200 g and 500 g in polythene bags and put in silver foil.

Evaluation

The hair should be easily washable with water. After washing:
1. The hair should be free from the shampoo.
2. Free from grease and dirt.
3. No itching on the scalp.
4. No irritation in the eyes or any other discomfort.
5. The hair should neither get decolourised nor loose original glossiness and softness.

MISCELLANEOUS

Herbal Pomades and Brilliantines

Pomades are the residues of floral extracts left over wax layers after the extraction of perfume by effleurage process. These are made from herbal hair oil by emulsification with 20% of water phase. These products help in managing the hair with ease.

Brilliantines are hair grooming preparation to add sheen to the hair and better manageability. Both solid and liquid brilliantines are available.

Formulations

Table 3.30

Solid brilliantine			Liquid brilliantine		
S. No.	Ingredient	%	S. No.	Ingredient	Parts
1.	Herbal hair oil	80	1.	Herbal hair oil	75
2.	Ethyl myristate	4	2.	Almond oil	20
3.	Castor oil	10	3.	Beeswax	5
4.	Stearic acid	2			
5.	Beeswax	3			
6.	Lanolin	1			
7.	Colour	QS			
8.	Perfume	QS			

Manufacturing of Brilliantine

All the ingredients are heated up to 65°C and filtered to give a transparent solution. The solid brilliantine solidifies into a translucent solid mass, when this liquid is cooled to 45°C.

Table 3.31

Pomades		
S. No.	Ingredient	%
1.	Herbal hair oil	80
2.	Beeswax	5
3.	Cetyl alcohol	3
4.	Water	12
6.	Perfume	QS
7.	Preservatives	QS
8.	Colour	QS

Manufacturing of Pomade

All the ingredients are heated at 70°C and stirred for half an hour till the liquid congeals to semisolid.

Quality Control

Uniform specific gravity and good spreadability.

Packing and Storage

Packed in HDPE containers and stored away from light and heat.

Evaluation

Manageability and comfort in grooming of the hair.

Antidandruff Products

An antidandruff application is meant to take care of alopaecia, damage caused by dandruff on the scalp and to prevent hair loss due to dandruff and any other incidental discomfort on the scalp like itching, etc.

Formulation

Table 3.32

S. No.	Ingredient	%
1.	Coconut oil	75
2.	Til oil	2
3.	Urtica diocca	5
4.	Mara manjal	5
5.	*Conscinium fenestratum*	5
6.	Datura metel leaves	8

Manufacturing

The above mixed plant extracts are boiled in coconut oil and til oil mixed in the ratio 70 : 30 and decanted after all the extracts are extracted by the oil base. The oil is dried over anhydrous calcium chloride or anhydrous sodium sulphate and put in the sun for one week till it is dry and free from moisture.

Quality Control

Clarity and specific gravity, non-greasy.

Packing and Storage

Packed in unit packs of 100 ml polypet or glass bottles and stored away from light and heat.

Evaluation

Adherence to the scalp, should make the scalp free from scales, itching and prevent loss of hair.

Anti-lice Products

The purpose of this product is to prevent lice on the head and the damage caused by head lice.

Formulation

Table 3.33

S. No.	Ingredient	%
1.	Coconut oil	70
2.	Til oil	15
3.	*Albizzia lebek*	5
4.	*Anona squamosa*—leaves	5
5.	*Anona squamosa*—seeds	5

Manufacturing

The above mixed plant extracts are boiled in coconut oil and til oil mixed in the ratio 70 : 30 and decanted after all the extracts are extracted by the oil base. The oil is dried over anhydrous calcium chloride or anhydrous sodium sulphate and put in the sun for one week till it is dry and free from moisture.

Quality Control

All the herbal extracts should get transferred into oil phase and the oil should be a transparent clear liquid.

Packing and Storage

Packed in unit packs of 100 ml glass or HDP bottles and stored away from sunlight.

Evaluation

The scalp and hair should be completely free of lice and knits of lice after 4 weeks of application on the head.

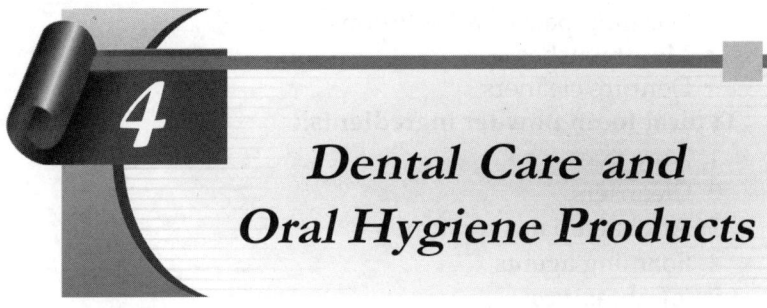

4

Dental Care and
Oral Hygiene Products

Oral hygiene products are used for keeping the teeth, gums and the oral cavity clean. The health of an individual is reflected through sparkling teeth, dazzling white colour and tight teeth and gums. In order to maintain healthy teeth, certain products are introduced in the market for oral cavity and mouth. Mouthwashes and gargling solutions, made out of astringent and antibacterial anti-inflammatory herbs are selected to serve the purpose. Tooth powders and pastes are for cleansing the teeth by removing the dental plaque and tartar and for keeping the oral cavity fresh.

ORAL CAVITY

Along with vital organs like heart, kidney and liver, gastro-intestinal tract (GIT) is also an important system in the body. The GIT starts with the oral cavity. GIT and oral cavity are the most vital organs and they have a lot of impact on the functioning of other vital organs.

Oral cavity can never be kept sterile. However, the density of microorganisms can be controlled. Hence, oral hygiene products, e.g. tooth powders and toothpastes help in removing tartar and plaque of teeth while mouthwashes and gargling solutions take care of the oral cavity.

Relevant oral hygiene products are of different types as under:
- Tooth powders
- Toothpastes
- Tartar removers

- Gargling packs and solutions
- Mouthwashes
- Denture cleaners

Typical tooth powder ingredients:

1. Abrasives
2. Cleansers
3. Antibacterial compounds
4. Foaming agents

List of abrasives:

1. Calcium carbonate
2. Calcium diphosphate
3. Calcium triphosphate
4. Sodium fluoride
5. *Sepia officinalis* powder
6. Silica gel siliceous earth
7. Magnesium aluminium silicate
8. Celite
9. Kieselguhr
10. Calcium carbonate
11. Sodium chloride
12. Hard soap powder
13. Charcoal powder

Flavouring agents:

1. Peppermint oil/spearmint oil
2. Wintergreen oil
3. Cinnamon oil
4. Clove oil
5. Anise oil
6. Gaultheria oil
7. Dill oil
8. Nutmeg oil
9. Fennel oil
10. Thymol
11. Anethol
12. Menthol
13. *Mentha arvensis*
14. *Mentha piperita*

List of sweeteners:

1. Glycerin
2. Sorbitol
3. Liquid glucose
4. Saccharin
5. Sodium cyclamate
6. Stevia powder

List of binders:

1. CMC
2. Sodium alginate
3. Gum karaya

Table 4.1: List of plants used in dental care and oral hygiene preparations

S. No.	Herb (Botanical name)	Parts used	Property
1.	Acacia arabica (Fig. 4.1)	Stem bark	Astringent, gum tightening
2.	Achyranthes aspera (Fig. 4.2)	Entire plant	Toothache
3.	Anacyclus pyrethrum (Fig. 4.3)	Roots	Toothache
4.	Azadirachta indica (Fig. 4.4)	Stem bark	Antibacterial
5.	Cressa cretica (Fig. 4.5)	Roots	Antiseptic
6.	Ficus benghalensis (Fig. 4.6)	Roots	Gum tightening
7.	Gaultheria procumbens (Fig. 4.7)	Leaves	Flavouring agent
8.	Mentha piperita (Fig. 4.8)	Oil	Flavouring, freshening
9.	Mimusops elengi (Fig. 4.9)	Fruit rind	Toothache, gargling
10.	Pongamia glabra (Fig. 4.10)	Bark	Antiseptic
11.	Psidium guajava (Fig. 4.11)	Leaves	Astringent
12.	Prunus amygdalus (Fig. 4.12)	Root bark	Tartar remover
13.	Sapindus mukorossi (Fig. 4.13)	Fruits	Cleansing
14.	Spilanthes acmella (Fig. 4.14)	Leaves, fruits	Toothache, gum infection
15.	Spilanthes calva (Fig. 4.15)	Flowers	Flavouring agent
16.	Spinifex squarrosus (Fig. 4.16)	Entire plant	Abrasive
17.	Syzygium aromaticum (Fig. 4.17)	Buds	Toothache
18.	Terminalia chebula (Fig. 4.18)	Stem bark	Astringent
19.	Zanthoxylum armatum (Fig. 4.19)	Leaves	Flavouring agent

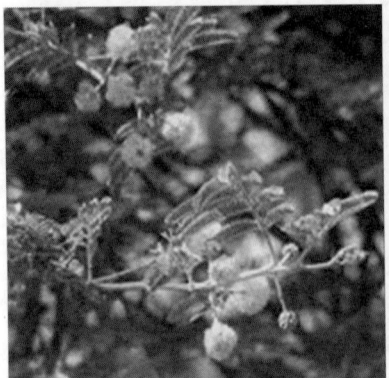

Fig. 4.1: *Acacia arabica*

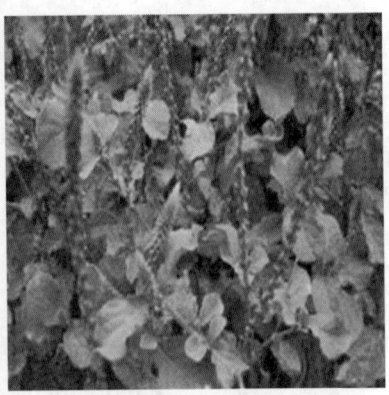

Fig. 4.2: *Achyranthes aspera*

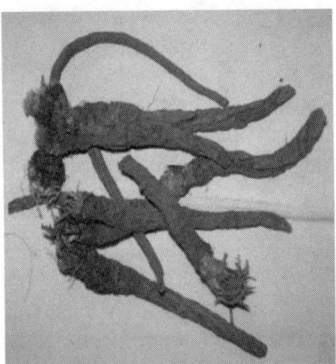

Fig. 4.3: *Anacyclus pyrethrum*

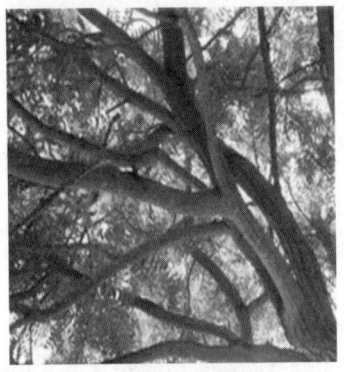

Fig. 4.4: *Azadirachta indica*

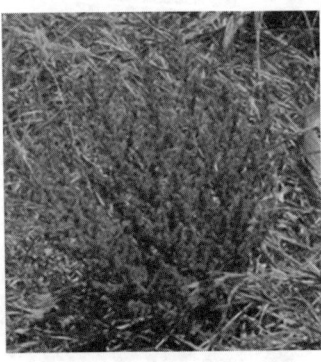

Fig. 4.5: *Cressa cretica*

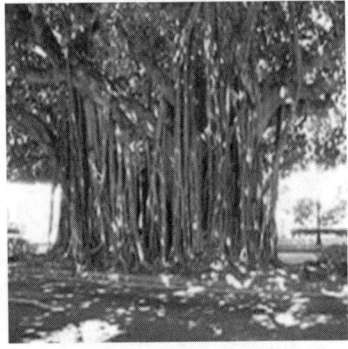

Fig. 4.6: *Ficus benghalensis*

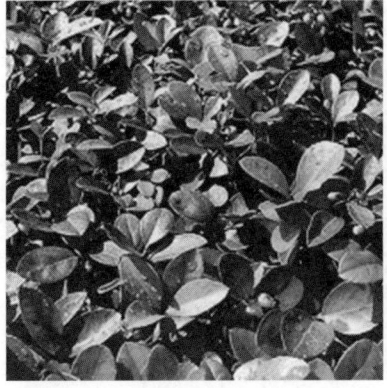

Fig. 4.7: *Gaultheria procumbens*

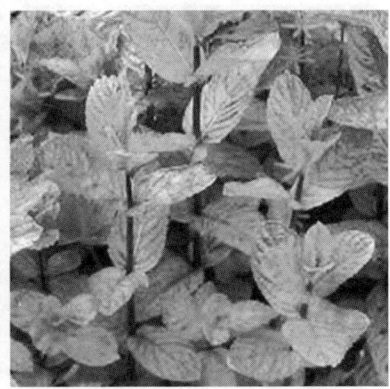

Fig. 4.8: *Mentha piperita*

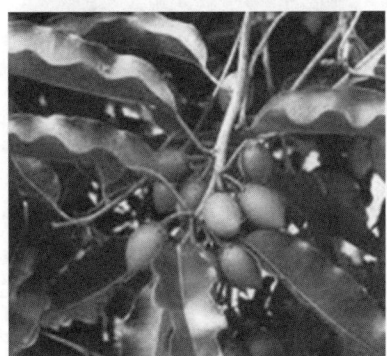

Fig. 4.9: *Mimusops elengi*

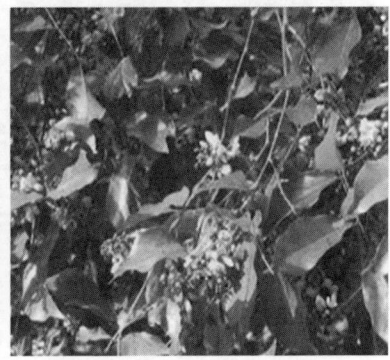

Fig. 4.10: *Pongamia glabra*

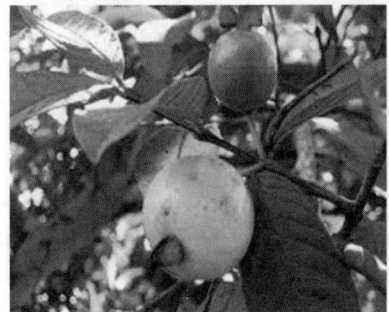

Fig. 4.11: *Psidium guajava*

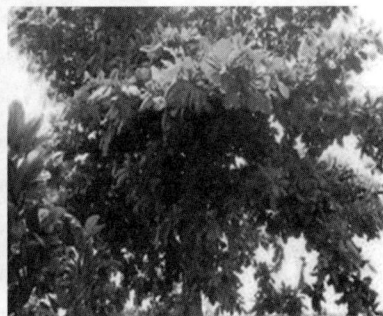

Fig. 4.12: *Prunus amygdalus*

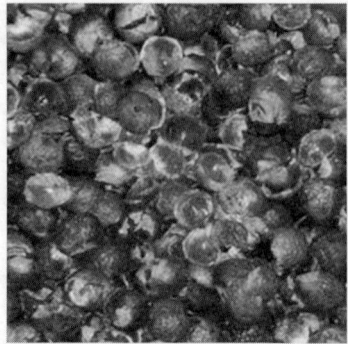

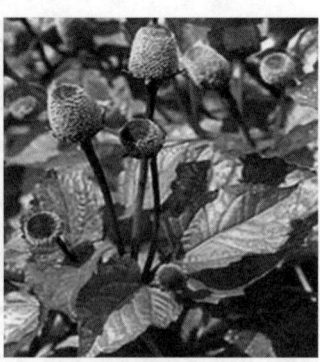

Fig. 4.13: *Sapindus mukorossi*

Fig. 4.14: *Spilanthes acmella*

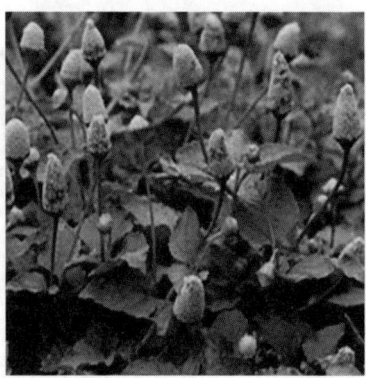

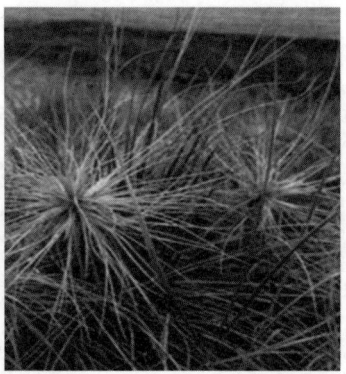

Fig. 4.15: *Spilanthes calva*

Fig. 4.16: *Spinifex squarrosus*

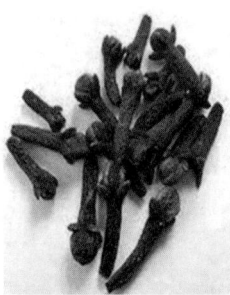

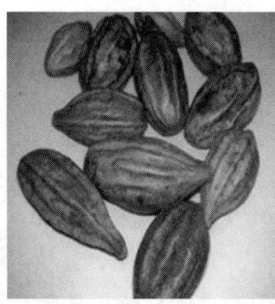

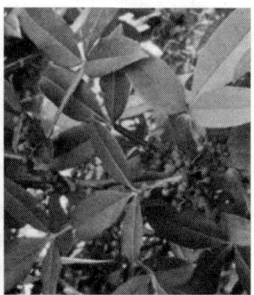

Fig. 4.17: *Syzygium aromaticum*

Fig. 4.18: *Terminalia chebula*

Fig. 4.19: *Zanthoxylum armatum*

TOOTH POWDER/PIGS

The traditional practice in India to clean the teeth is by chewing twigs of neem and karangia. Chewing exercises teeth, cleans and keeps the mouth fresh. Then came tooth powders.

Traditionally tender plant twigs of neem, karangia, *Achyranthes aspera* were chewed and then used as a brush in conjunction with tooth powder to clean the teeth. Later on tooth pastes were developed from powder in order to make powders more consumer acceptable and convenient.

The discomfort and disadvantage of tooth powder is that because of dusting it may cause choking and also leave stains.

Formulations
Oldest Formula
Table 4.2

Base			Herbal powder mix		
S. No.	*Ingredient*	*%*	*S. No.*	*Ingredient*	*Parts*
1.	Salt	3	1.	*Azadirachta indica*—bark	5
2.	Ash or burnt cowdung cakes	40	2.	*Acacia arabica*—bark	2
3.	Neem bark powder	5	3.	*Pongamia glabra*—bark	3
4.	Burnt soapnut fruits powder	10			
5.	Calcium carbonate	25			
6.	Activated charcoal	7			
7.	Herbal powder mix	10			
8.	Foaming agent (hard soap powder)	QS			

Table 4.3

Base			Herbal powder mix		
S. No.	*Ingredient*	*%*	*S. No.*	*Ingredient*	*Parts*
1.	Calcium carbonate	50	1.	*Mimusops elengi* fruit bark	2.5
2.	Celite	30	2.	*Azadirachta indica*—bark	2.5
3.	Sodium chloride	5	3.	*Acacia arabica*—bark	2.5
4.	Hard soap powder	5	4.	*Pongamia glabra*—bark	2.5
5.	Herbal powder mix	10			
6.	Flavouring agent	QS			

Flavour—Essential Oil Mixture

Table 4.4

S. No.	Ingredient	Parts
1.	Cinnamon oil	2
2	Clove oil	2
3.	Peppermint/spearmint oil	2
4.	Neem, karangia oils	4

Special Tooth Powder

Table 4.5

Base			Herbal powder mix		
S. No.	Ingredient	%	S. No.	Ingredient	Parts
1.	Charcoal	20	1.	*Azadirachta indica*—bark	2
2.	Cuttle fish bone powder	55	2.	*Pongamia glabra*—bark	2
3.	Sodium fluoride	5	3.	*Mimusops elengi*—bark	2
4.	Soap powder	5			
5.	Magnesium carbonate	5			
6.	Herbal powder mix	10			
7.	Flavouring agent	QS			

Levigated wood charcoal is the base and bodying agent for this tooth powder.

Cocoa Tooth Powder

Table 4.6

S. No.	Ingredient	%
1.	Cocoa powder	10
2.	Calcium carbonate	70
3.	Magnesium carbonate	5
4.	Colloidal silica	5
5.	Aluminium hydroxide	10
6.	Flavouring agent	QS

This powder has an extra property of inhibiting plaque formation apart from pleasant taste in the mouth.

Table 4.7

Base			Herbal powder mix		
S. No.	Ingredient	%	S. No.	Ingredient	Parts
1.	Calcium carbonate	70	1.	Acacia arabica	5
2.	Dicalcium phosphate	15	2.	Azadirachta indica—bark	5
3.	Magnesium carbonate	5	3.	Cressa cretica	5
4.	Herbal powder mix	10			
5.	Flavouring agent	QS			

Table 4.8

Base			Herbal powder mix		
S. No.	Ingredient	%	S. No.	Ingredient	Parts
1.	Calcium carbonate	50	1.	Achyranthes aspera	5
2.	Clay	20	2.	Anacyclus pyrethrum	5
3.	Magnesium carbonate	5			
4.	Dicalcium phosphate	15			
5.	Herbal powder mix	10			
6.	Flavouring agent	QS			

Table 4.9

Base			Herbal powder mix		
S. No.	Ingredient	%	S. No.	Ingredient	Parts
1.	Calcium carbonate	60	1.	Achyranthes aspera	2
2.	Dicalcium phosphate	10	2.	Azadirachta indica—bark	2
3.	Magnesium carbonate	5	3.	Pongamia glabra—bark	2
4.	Celite	15			
5.	Herbal powder mix	10			
6.	Flavouring agent	QS			

Manufacturing

All the ingredients are powdered and passed through 80 mesh and blended with mixed magnesium carbonate and flavouring agent(s).

The essential oils are thoroughly mixed with magnesium carbonate and transferred to the base along with herbal powder mix and finally transferred into a double cone blender, to obtain thorough uniform mixing.

Due to herbal powder, there is a tendency of clogging, as the herbal powder can absorb moisture from the atmosphere. To improve the flowability, a slurry is made with a small quantity of detergent, followed by drying and granulating and sieving the granulated slurry into required particle size, generally 60/100 mesh.

Quality Control

Specific gravity, viscosity, non-gritty texture. The powder should pass through 80/100 mesh. Uniformity in mixing of both herbal powders and essential oils.

Packing and Storage

Tooth powders are packed either in metal or plastic bottles and stored away from moisture.

Evaluation

It should clean the teeth from plaque and dental tartar without damaging the enamel coat of the teeth. It should not stain the teeth. It should keep the oral cavity fresh and mask any bad breath in the oral cavity.

TOOTHPASTE

These are pastes meant for cleaning teeth from tartar and plaque.

Table 4.10

Base			Flavouring agent		
S. No.	Ingredient	%	S. No.	Ingredient	Parts
1.	Herbal tooth powder	65	1.	Peppermint oil	2
2.	Detergent (neutral)	3	2.	Wintergreen oil	2
3.	Sodium lauroyl sarcosinate	2	3.	Cinnamon oil	2
4.	Sodium mono-flurophosphate	10			
5.	Celite	15			
6.	Sweetener—glycerin sorbitol	2			
7.	Flavouring agent	3			
8.	Sodium alginate	QS			

Manufacturing

30% of sodium flurophosphate, celite, sorbitol, detergent are mixed under vacuum and blended with a portion of sorbitol and glycerin, water with sodium alginate and made into a solution. The mixing and stirring is continued for 4 hrs. Then rest of glycerin and sorbitol are mixed with the blended mass, stirring is continued under vacuum for another four hours.

Table 4.11

Base			Flavouring agent		
S. No.	Ingredient	%	S. No.	Ingredient	Parts
1.	Herbal tooth powder	60	1.	Clove oil	2
2.	Silica fine	5	2.	Cinnamon oil	2
3.	Lactose	5	3.	Karanjia oil	2
4.	Foaming agent	5	4.	Menthol	2
5.	Burnt soapnut fruit powder	5			
6.	Cuttle fish bone powder	10			
7.	Magnesium carbonate	5			
8.	Sorbitol	5			
9.	Flavouring agent	QS			
10.	Water	QS			
11.	Sodium alginate	QS			

Manufacturing

All the powders from 1 to 6 in the above formula are mixed with the foaming agent and lactose, thoroughly. Then sodium alginate suspension is added with flavouring agent and mixed thoroughly once again, kept for 24 hrs in storage tank to observe any change in the viscosity, before packing into tubes and sealing.

Table 4.12

Base			Flavouring agent		
S. No.	Ingredient	%	S. No.	Ingredient	Parts
1.	Herbal tooth powder	70	1.	Clove oil	2
2.	Detergent	3	2.	Cinnamon oil	2
3.	Flavouring agent	3	3.	Peppermint oil	2
4.	Water	20			
5.	Sweetener	4			
6.	Glycerin	QS			
7.	Sodium alginate	QS			

Table 4.13

Base			Herbal extracts mix		
S. No.	Ingredient	%	S. No.	Ingredient	Parts
1.	Calcium carbonate	55	1.	Clove extract	5
2.	Kieselguhr	5	2.	Pongamia glabra	5
3.	Magnesium carbonate	5		bark extract	
4.	Water	20	3.	Azadirachta indica	5
5.	Glycerin	5		bark extract	
6.	Sorbitol	5	4.	Gum arabica extract	5
7.	Soap powder	5			
8.	Sodium alginate	QS			
9.	Sweetener—sodium cyclamate	QS			

Manufacturing

All the herbal extracts, gum arabica, glycerin, sorbitol and water are all stirred for 4 hrs under vacuum. Then the powders, calcium carbonate, magnesium carbonate, flavouring oils are also added and the mixing is continued for another two hours. Kept aside for observing stability for about a week, before packing.

Table 4.14

S. No.	Ingredient	%		S. No.	Ingredient	Parts
Base				**Herbal extracts mix**		
1.	Calcium carbonate	60		1.	Gum Arabica—bark	5
2.	Celite	10		2.	*Pongamia glabra*—bark	5
3.	Magnesium carbonate	7		3.	*Azadirachta indica*—bark	5
4.	Detergent (soap powder)	3				
5.	Sorbitol	5				
6.	Water	15				
7.	Sodium alginate	QS				
8.	Flavouring (cinnamon oil, clove oil)	QS				

Table 4.15

S. No.	Ingredient	%
1.	Herbal tooth powder	10
2.	Calcium phosphate	5
3.	Calcium carbonate	49.8
4.	Magnesium aluminium silicate	10
5.	Sodium saccharin	0.2
6.	Sodium cocoyl sulphate	5
7.	Sodium monoglyceride sulphate	5
8.	Sodium lauryl sulphate	3
9.	Titanium dioxide	2
10.	Stannous fluoride aluminium silicate	5
11.	Sorbitol	5
12.	Water	QS
13.	Flavouring agent	QS

Manufacturing

The powders are mixed thoroughly in a blender and then sorbitol, glycerol and water with herbal extracts mix is added to the powders along with sodium alginate solution and mixed in a Hovert mixer to get a uniform mass and free from any clogs or lumps. The whole mass is kept in a storage tank for 48 hrs and then filled in the tubes.

Quality Control

The paste should be uniform, without any clogs or lumps to maintain the uniform viscosity of about 70,000 to 1,00,000 cps throughout the shelf life. It should cleanse the teeth, leaving freshness in the mouth. No leaking of liquid or separation. Neither should it run off the packed tube nor cause difficulty in coming out smoothly, when it is squeezed from the tube. It should not harden on standing.

Packing and Storage

Tooth pastes are packed in collapsible tubes, either metal or plastic and stored away from light and heat in a dry place.

Evaluation

Cleansing, dental plaque removing or making the teeth free from dental plaque and tartar and polishing. It should not alter or discolour the teeth and impart any damage to the enamel coat of the teeth. It should leave the mouth with lingering flavour of the essential oils, masking any bad breath of the mouth.

TARTAR REMOVER

Tartar and its incrustations are dissolved by the herbal powder mix. Thus, it acts as a tartar remover and a polishing product.

Formulations

Table 4.16

S. No.	Ingredient	%	S. No.	Ingredient	Parts
1.	Sileous earth	80	1.	Cocoa powder	10
2.	Celite powder	5	2.	*Prunus amygdalus*	2
3.	Soap powder	2		tree root bark	
4.	Magnesium carbonate	5			
5.	Menthol	1			
6.	Clove oil	1			
7.	Cinnamon oil	1			
8.	Herbal powder mix	5			
9.	Preservatives	QS			

Dental Film Preventor

Table 4.17

S. No.	Ingredient	Parts
1.	Calcium carbonate	70
2.	Magnesium carbonate	5
3.	Celite	20
4.	Clove oil	2
5.	Cinnamon oil	2
6.	Sweetener—stevia powder	1

Manufacturing

All the ingredients are thoroughly blended and bottled in either PVC or glass bottles.

GARGLING POWDERS IN PACKS

They are used for keeping the oral cavity anti-bacterial after gargling. Gargling solutions made out of herbal powders and water are useful in taking care of the oral mouth, making it free from any inflammation, pain or bleeding of gums and tooth cavities. These are generally used whenever there is either a throat or gum or teeth infection in the oral cavity.

Formulations

Table 4.18

S. No.	Ingredient	Parts
1.	Terminalia chebula—powder	5
2.	Alum	5
3.	Punica granatum—powder	5
4.	Azadirachta indica—powder	5

Manufacturing

Gargles are prepared by adding the powder pack in warm water in the ratio 1:10. The solution is decanted, and bottled and stored away from light. About 10 ml solution is used for gargling by keeping in the mouth for 10 minutes with thorough rinsing before throwing it out.

Quality Control

1. Specific gravity and
2. Free from suspended matter.

Packing and Storage

Packed in volumes of 200 or 500 ml in PVC or glass bottles with air tight lids and stored away from light and heat.

Evaluation

After gargling with the solution, the mouth should be free from infection, inflammation, bleeding and pain if any.

MOUTHWASH

Oral hygiene products are dental care products to keep the dental structure intact, free from infections, protecting the enamel and the cavity, gums, etc. and also from bad breath. Gargles and mouthwashes are used after cleaning the oral cavity, leaving it fresh and free from bad breath, with tingling effect. Mouthwashes are mostly used to mask any foul odor of oral cavity and also to keep it fresh.

Formulations

Herbal Mouthwash

Table 4.19

S. No.	Ingredient	%
1.	Thymol	1
2.	Peppermint oil	2
3.	Wintergreen oil	2
4.	Alcohol	3
5.	Water	80
6.	Glycerin	2
7.	Liquid glucose	5
8.	Tejphal	5
9.	Colour	QS

Table 4.20

S. No.	Ingredient	%
1.	Alcohol	5
2.	Water	90
3.	Spearmint oil	2
4.	*Spinifex squarrosus* extract	3
5.	Colour	QS
6.	Cinnamon oil	QS
7.	Clove oil	QS

Antiseptic Mouthwash

Table 4.21

S. No.	Ingredient	%
1.	Water	85
2.	*Pongamia glabra* extract	5
3.	*Cressa cretica* extract	5
4.	Glycerin	5
5.	Colour	QS
6.	Gaultheria oil	QS
7.	Clove oil	QS

Table 4.22

S. No.	Ingredient	%
1.	Stevia	2
2.	*Mimusops elangi* fruit bark extract	3
3.	Alcohol	5
4.	Water	90
5.	Colour—green or orange or blue	QS
6.	Anise oil	QS
7.	Clove oil	QS
8.	Peppermint oil	QS
9.	Menthol	QS

Manufacturing

All the ingredients in the formulae given are mixed thoroughly and filtered after shaking with celite for 5 minutes.

Quality Control

A transparent crystal clear liquid with 1.1 specific gravity and reproducible refractive index from batch to batch.

Packing and Storage

Packed in 200 or 500 ml PVC or glass bottles with air tight lids and stored away from light and heat.

Evaluation

After using the solution, the mouth should be free from any bad odor.

DENTURE CLEANERS

A suspension of montmorillonite with surfactant and herbal extracts and dicalcium phosphate with 0.1% clove oil or menthol are useful in cleaning the denture. The denture is cleaned with this suspension in conjunction with a soft tooth brush and then immersed in potable water overnight before using next day.

Formulations

Table 4.23

S. No.	Ingredient	%
1.	Dicalcium phosphate	10
2.	Montmorillonite	10
3.	Surfactant	2
4.	Water	73
5.	Pudina leaf extract	5
6.	Clove oil	QS
7.	Menthol	QS

Table 4.24

S. No.	Ingredient	%
1.	Dicalcium phosphate	5
2.	Montmorillonite	5
3.	Kieselguhr	5
4.	Zinc chloride	5
5.	Distilled water	75
6.	*Achyranthes aspera* extract	5
7.	Flavouring agent	QS

Manufacturing

All the ingredients are mixed and stirred with 0.2% surfactant for 2 hrs, kept overnight and packed after 24 hrs.

Quality Control

1. The suspension should be uniform dispersible, free flowing.
2. Should cleanse and polish the denture.

Packing and Storage

The solution is bottled in 500 ml quantity either in glass or PVC bottles and stored away from light and heat.

Evaluation

The denture should be free from any embedded particles in between the denture structure and any other deposits.

Index

Reader's Notes

Reader's Notes

_____

_____

_____

_____

_____

_____

_____

_____

_____

_____

_____

_____

_____

_____

_____

_____

_____

_____

_____

_____

_____

_____

_____

_____

_____

_____

Reader's Notes

_____

_____

_____

_____

_____

_____

_____

_____

_____

_____

_____

_____

_____

_____

_____

_____

_____

_____

_____

_____

_____

_____

_____

_____

_____

Reader's Notes

_____

_____

_____

_____

_____

_____

_____

_____

_____

_____

_____

_____

_____

_____

_____

_____

_____

_____

_____

_____

_____

_____

_____

_____